managing
menopause
with diet, vitamins and herbs

An Essential Guide for the
Peri and Post Menopausal Years

Leslie Beck RD

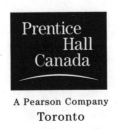

Prentice
Hall
Canada

A Pearson Company
Toronto

Canadian Cataloguing in Publication Data

Beck, Leslie (Leslie C.)
  Managing menopause with diet, vitamins and herbs: an essential guide for the peri- and
post-menopause years

Includes index.
ISBN 0-13-017966-3

1. Menopause – Complications – Alternative treatment. 2. Menopause – Nutritional aspects.
I. Title.

RG186.B424 2000   618.1'7506   C00-930175-5

ISBN 0-13-017966-3

Editorial Director, Trade Division: Andrea Crozier
Copy Editor: Sibylle Preuschat
Production Editor: Jodi Lewchuk
Art Direction: Mary Opper
Interior Design: Gary Beelik
Production Manager: Kathrine Pummell
Page Layout: Janet Zanette

1 2 3 4 5 WC 04 03 02 01 00

Printed and bound in Canada.

This publication contains the opinions and ideas of its author and is designed to provide useful
advice in regard to the subject matter covered. The author and publisher are not engaged in
rendering health or other professional services in this publication. This publication is not
intended to provide a basis for action in particular circumstances without consideration by a
competent professional. The author and publisher expressly disclaim any responsibility for any
liability or risk, personal or otherwise, which is incurred as a consequence, directly or indirectly,
of the use and application of any of the contents of this book.

Visit the Prentice Hall Canada Web site! Send us your comments, browse our catalogues, and
more. **www.phcanada.com.**

Prentice
Hall
Canada

A Pearson Company

To my mother and my female clients.
Your questions, your openness and your trust in me
made writing this book possible.

contents

APPENDICES

Introduction

If you are a woman in your 40s, 50s, or 60s, this book is a must have. Perhaps you are experiencing changes in your monthly menstrual cycle, not to mention uncomfortable physical symptoms. Or maybe you are a woman in your post-menopausal years and you're concerned about protecting your bones and your heart. Whether you are perimenopausal or post-menopausal, whether you are taking hormones or not, this book will help you make smart changes to your diet, add the right vitamin and mineral supplements to your daily routine, and choose the most appropriate herbal remedies for your symptoms. In short, this book will help you stay healthy and feel better, the natural way, during your menopausal years.

As a professional nutritionist (Registered Dietitian), I have been giving women and men advice on diet and supplements for the past 12 years. I assess my clients' diet, medical history, and lifestyle and then develop customized nutrition plans that will help them reach their goals. Because my private practice is located in the heart of downtown Toronto's financial district, many of my clients are baby boomers—women and men who are taking charge of their health care. They want to eat to stay healthy into their later years, to have plenty of energy, and to avoid taking medications if possible.

During the past five years, I have been getting an increasing number of requests for nutrition advice regarding menopause. If a woman comes to see me because she wants to lose weight or lower her cholesterol levels, she invariably also asks me what she can do for her hot flashes, or what supplements she should be taking in light of her most recent bone density test, or how she should eat to help reduce her risk of breast cancer.

Today in Canada almost 3.5 million women are between the ages of 40 and 54, the phase of life when levels of certain hormones are changing and dwindling. As baby boomers get older, the number of women in this situation will only increase. What's more, the number of women entering the post-menopausal years will increase by 50 percent over the next 10 years. The demand for advice will continue to grow.

As women decide to prepare their bodies for hormonal changes and the health risks that ensue, many are frustrated by the lack of information available to help them do this. Books on diet and nutrition are lacking and most doctors don't have the answers because they aren't trained in nutrition or alternative therapies. And even if they are knowledgeable, doctors don't have the time to assess your food intake and develop a nutrition plan for you. If you want sound advice that's tailored to your lifestyle, a visit to a qualified nutritionist is in order. Registered dietitians are university-educated experts who are trained in how nutrition affects both health and disease.

I realized that there was a great need for this book not only when I considered the large numbers of women entering menopause, but also when I could not find one book on menopause that covered diet, nutrition, and supplemental herbs in depth. If you walk into a bookstore, you will find plenty of books on menopause, but most don't mention nutrition. And the few books out there that do discuss diet only skim the surface when it comes to vitamin or herbal supplements. In writing this book, I want to help you understand why certain foods, supplements, and herbs may help you feel better and be healthier, and how to incorporate them into your daily routines.

Managing Menopause with Diet, Vitamins and Herbs is an essential guide for any woman who wants to:

- Ease the symptoms of perimenopause, including hot flashes, insomnia, mood swings, sexual changes, and more.
- Lose weight or prevent weight gain associated with lifestyle habits, advancing age, or hormone replacement therapy.
- Reduce her risk of breast cancer, heart disease, and osteoporosis, health problems most often experienced in the post-menopausal years.

THE TERMINOLOGY OF MENOPAUSE

The signs and symptoms associated with the beginning of menopause occur over a period of time, called the perimenopause. This word literally means "around menopause." The perimenopause can begin up to 10 years before menopause, when hormonal changes start to happen. For many women, the first sign of perimenopause is an erratic menstrual cycle—skipped, lighter, or shorter periods. The hallmark of this countdown to menopause is fluctuating levels of the female hormones estrogen and progesterone. Estrogen highs can bring on PMS-like symptoms including mood swings, fluid retention, and headaches, whereas estrogen lows promise hot flashes, vaginal dryness, and forgetfulness. While perimenopause can start in the late thirties, most women begin noticing symptoms in their forties.

You're considered to have reached menopause when a year has passed since your last period. The average age at which a Canadian women reaches menopause is 51. It's at this time that women enter the post-menopause, the phase of life in which the risk of developing heart disease, osteoporosis, and breast cancer increases.

Hormones and your menstrual cycle

In order to understand what's happening to your body during perimenopause, it helps to know how your hormones normally act during the childbearing years. During the early part of your monthly cycle, your ovaries produce estrogen. Your brain responds to this increasing estrogen level by telling your pituitary gland to release follicle stimulating hormone (FSH) and luteinizing hormone (LH). These two hormones, in turn, act on your ovaries. FSH causes egg follicles to develop and release estrogen. When circulating estrogen rises to a critical level, the pituitary gland releases a surge of LH. This influx of LH causes ovulation by telling the follicle to release a mature egg. The empty egg follicle turns into something called the corpus luteum, a gland that produces progesterone after ovulation. During the last 14 days of your menstrual cycle, progesterone prepares your body for pregnancy by thickening the lining of your uterus. If conception does not occur, the corpus luteum becomes smaller, estrogen and progesterone levels fall, and your uterine lining is shed, resulting in your period. Lower levels of estrogen and progesterone signal your pituitary to release FSH and LH and the cycle begins anew.

Hormonal changes during perimenopause

As you get older, your supply of eggs and follicles dwindles. When there are fewer follicles, your ovaries produce less estrogen. Lower levels of estrogen and progesterone tell your pituitary gland that it's time to release FSH and then LH. But now your ovaries are unable to respond to FSH and LH. They can't produce much estrogen and release an egg, and as a result your brain keeps on telling your pituitary gland to make your ovaries ovulate. So your pituitary gland keeps on releasing more and more FSH. You'll read in Chapter 1 how this constant production of FSH can trigger hot flashes. Also, with no egg being released from your ovary, there's no corpus luteum and consequently, no progesterone secretion. Without progesterone your body won't shed its uterine lining and you'll miss a period. With overall lower levels of hormones, your periods will also become shorter and eventually they will cease.

The hormone replacement therapy dilemma

Should you take hormone replacement therapy (HRT)? That's certainly a question that every woman will be faced with at some point in her life. And if you're reading this book, chances are it will be sooner rather than later. While some of you are no doubt mulling this question over right now, many of you have already made your decision. And more than likely some of you have filled your prescription and taken the hormones, only to quit a short time later. Adherence to hormone replacement therapy is low. One survey of 2,500 post-menopausal American women done in 1982 revealed that 20 percent of women had stopped taking HRT within nine months of starting, due to fear of cancer or side effects. Another 10 percent used HRT off and on, while up to 30 percent never bothered to fill their prescription. A more recent study indicated that only 28 percent of American women over the age of 50 were taking HRT. Among the two-thirds who were non-users, 82 percent were menopausal.[1]

Most women take HRT to get relief for troublesome symptoms. I have a number of clients who find their hot flashes are unbearable and affect their productivity at the office—not to mention how self-conscious they become in a business meeting dominated by men. Other women find their mood swings take over and impact their family life. There's no question that short-term estrogen therapy alleviates these symptoms.

Many other women start on HRT after discussing their health risks with their family physician. It's clear that HRT lowers the risk of heart disease in post-menopausal women by 40 to 50 percent. And women who take hormones have higher bone density and a lower risk of bone fracture compared to women who don't use the drugs. So if you have a high risk of heart disease or osteoporosis, HRT may be a wise idea. Keep in mind, however, that its protective effects only last as long as you continue using it.

And unfortunately, HRT is not without risks. When taken for more than 5 to 10 years, HRT increases the risk of breast cancer. But that's assuming you can tolerate the side effects for such a period of time. Certain regimes cause bloating, nausea, weight gain, and breast soreness, frequently cited reasons for stopping the medication.

Using HRT is neither right nor wrong. It is a decision every woman must make based on her personal medical history and tolerance of perimenopausal symptoms. It's a decision that needs to be made in consultation with your doctor. And you should know that there are options. Taking hormone replacement by pill, cream, or patch can influence the potential for side effects. Changing the dosage can also make a difference. Depending on your body size, a lower daily dose may be able to eliminate side effects and offer as much protection against serious disease as a higher one. If you are taking HRT and finding it difficult to tolerate the side effects, or if you are finding it ineffective at relieving your symptoms, ask your doctor about your options.

How this book will help you if you don't take hormones

More and more Canadian women are seeking alternative approaches to HRT. Whether you are trying to ease hot flashes, manage mood swings, or prevent heart disease, this book gives you a step-by-step approach to changing your diet, adding vitamin and mineral supplements, and choosing helpful herbal remedies. All of my recommendations are based on scientific evidence—throughout the book, I translate the scientific findings into information that you can put into practice. If you choose not to take hormones, my advice and diet plans will help you:

- Ease or eliminate symptoms associated with perimenopause: hot flashes, night sweats, insomnia, depression, anxiety, forgetfulness, vaginal dryness, and heavy periods.
- Manage your weight throughout the menopausal years.
- Eat a diet that lowers your risk of developing breast cancer, coronary heart disease, and osteoporosis.

How this book will help you if you do take hormones

If you are currently using HRT, you'll learn that there are a number of things that you can do be doing at the same time to lower your chances of disease:

- Making certain dietary changes will help ease menopausal symptoms and may allow you to lower your HRT dose.
- Incorporating certain foods and supplements can give you more protection from osteoporosis and heart disease than that offered by hormones alone.

- Making dietary changes can help to prevent the weight gain often associated with hormone use.
- Eating right can increase your feeling of energy and well being.

HOW THIS BOOK IS ORGANIZED

It's time to begin learning and making positive lifestyle changes. I have divided my book into three parts: symptom relief, weight control, and disease risk reduction. That way, depending on what stage of menopause you're in and how it's affecting you, you can spend your time reading what's most important. I've also tried to make the information easy to read. In every chapter, I list my recommendations in three categories: dietary strategies, vitamins and minerals, and herbal remedies. And if you don't want to read about how a food, vitamin, or herb works in your body, you can skip ahead to the end of the chapter where I summarize my recommendations in "The Bottom Line" section. At the end of the book you'll find "Leslie's Total Nutrition Plan for the Menopausal Years" with modifications for weight loss. And all along the way, you'll find quotes from my clients, friends, and relatives, talking about their experiences of perimenopause and menopause—their words are proof that you're not alone.

I hope you enjoy this book and find it a useful guide to better nutrition.

Leslie Beck, RD
Toronto

managing your symptoms

"I suddenly have a hot flash. I know that I am beet red from the neck up and the perspiration is starting to run down my forehead. Someone suggests, 'It's very warm in here today,' and I am truly mortified. I have just broadcast to my younger male colleagues that I am menopausal!"

hot flashes and night sweats

"The strange thing about hot flashes is that you don't realize what they are until you start noticing that on a regular basis, you are the only one in the room perspiring from the heat."

I

Hot flashes are, without a doubt, the most commonly reported symptom of menopause—indeed, hot flashes are often the first sign that menopause is approaching. Between 60 and 85 percent of North American women experience hot flashes at some point during the perimenopausal or post-menopausal years. Ten to 15 percent of these women experience hot flashes so severe that they interfere with daily life. On average, hot flashes persist for two to three years, but in 50 percent of women who experience this symptom, they last for up to five years. A small group of women get hot flashes for periods of 15 years or longer, sometimes experiencing them into their 70s and 80s.

anatomy of a hot flash

Hot flashes vary considerably among women with respect to their frequency, intensity, and duration. A warning signal often precedes a hot flash. This signal may take the form of an "aura," similar to that experienced by migraine sufferers. The aura may manifest as pressure in the head, a headache, or a wave of nausea. A sensation of heat then starts in the head and neck and spreads to the torso, arms, and entire body. Sweating follows and is most intense in the upper body. Clothing may become soaked, particularly if hot flashes occur during sleep. Some women experience heart palpitations, dizziness, or feelings of tension and anxiety. Hot flashes, as I explain in more detail below, actually cool the body, and chills or shakes may follow the flash as a result of the drop in body temperature it has caused. The entire event can last anywhere from a few seconds to several minutes; it can then take up to an hour for the resultant chills to subside. I have some clients who experience hot flashes as often as one every hour, while others report as few as several per week. Hot flashes may disappear for months, only to return when you least expect them. Many women report that stressful events or warm temperatures or warm rooms aggravate hot flashes. Consuming caffeine and alcohol, or even eating a spicy meal, can trigger hot flashes in some women. Fortunately though, hot flashes usually resolve with age and as your body adjusts to the changes of the menopausal years.

Night sweats are another term for hot flashes that occur during sleep. Often nocturnal hot flashes can be severe enough to disrupt sleep and cause insomnia, fatigue, and irritability. Chapters 2 and 3 cover natural treatment of these symptoms.

To understand hot flashes better, let's take a closer look at the hormones involved.

HORMONES

A hormone is any chemical substance produced in the body that has a specific regulatory effect on the activity of certain cells or organs.

Estrogen

The term estrogen is a generic word for a group of female sex hormones, including estradiol, estriol, and estrone. You form estrogens in your ovaries, brain, and fatty tissues. At puberty, estrogen stimulates breast development and other female characteristics. Estrogen also stimulates the uterine lining (endometrium) to grow during the pre-ovulatory phase of the menstrual cycle, to prepare you for possible pregnancy.

Follicle stimulating hormone (FSH)

This hormone is produced by your pituitary gland, which is inside your brain. For the first 14 days of your menstrual cycle, FSH stimulates the follicles in your ovaries to produce estrogen. When estrogen levels have risen adequately, the pituitary gland turns off FSH production. After menopause, when your ovaries no longer respond to FSH, your blood levels of FSH stay high. During the perimenopausal years, your FSH levels can fluctuate.

Luteinizing hormone (LH)

This hormone is also produced in your pituitary gland, and like FSH, it acts on your ovaries. LH is released once your estrogen levels rise and FSH is turned off. When your level of LH is at its highest, your ovarian follicle releases an egg (ovulation).

Progesterone

Once you ovulate, your follicle (now called a *corpeus luteum*) produces progesterone in addition to estrogen. Progesterone acts to build up the uterine lining. When progesterone and estrogen levels drop, your body sheds its uterine lining by having a period, and your pituitary gland know that it's time to start releasing FSH once more.

WHAT CAUSES HOT FLASHES?

We are still trying to understand exactly what happens in the body to cause a hot flash. Hot flashes begin in the hypothalamus, the region of the brain that houses the body's temperature control centre. It decides that you are too hot (even though your body temperature is normal) and attempts to cool you down by increasing your heartbeat and sending more blood to your skin, especially the skin of your head and neck. As a result, blood vessels in your skin dilate, your skin flushes, and you sweat. The overall effect is that heat escapes from your body. Paradoxically, hot flashes are your body's way of cooling down—even though you don't need to. What might cause the hypothalamus to become confused about your actual temperature and trigger a hot flash?

As you enter the menopausal years, estrogen production drops and ovulation begins becoming irregular, and then comes to a stop altogether. Without enough estrogen, your body can't thicken the lining of your uterus. You'll get irregular periods and eventually, your periods will cease. Without ovulation, progesterone levels fall. But remember, low estrogen and progesterone levels tell your pituitary that it's time to release FSH and then LH. But now your ovaries are no longer able to respond to FSH and LH. They can't produce much estrogen or release an egg, so your hypothalamus keeps telling your pituitary gland to make your ovaries ovulate. As a result, your pituitary gland keeps releasing more and more FSH (that's why FSH levels are high during menopause). Your hypothalamus is so busy constantly signaling your pituitary gland, that its temperature control centre can malfunction, setting off a hot flash even though temperature adjustment isn't needed. Experts also believe that a drop in estrogen levels may trigger your hypothalamus and as a result, your body's temperature control system malfunctions.

COPING WITH HOT FLASHES

It is interesting to note that hot flashes don't exist in some cultures. In the Japanese language, for instance, there is no word for "hot flash." Women in traditional cultures generally make the transition into the menopausal years experiencing very few, or none, of the distressing symptoms suffered by women in our western culture. Research indicates that women in these cultures tend to view menopause as a healthy, natural part of aging, rather than as an unwanted medical condition. And researchers have learned that there is definitely a link between a society's attitude towards menopause and the symptoms commonly experienced by women in that society. With today's focus on beauty, sexiness, and thinness, many women find themselves at odds with menopause. They are afraid that menopause means becoming "old" and "useless." I remember vividly listening to one client as she described her anxieties about menopause as a fear of "becoming old," "becoming fat," and "knitting all day long." It seems common for women to be afraid they won't be valued by society after they pass through menopause.

So how does all this relate to my original question—what can we do about hot flashes? Well, we can start by learning from women in Eastern and other traditional cultures and adopting a more accepting and respecting attitude towards our bodies' natural life cycle changes—and we can pick up other hints from them as well. Japanese women eat plenty of soy foods and fish and very few high-fat animal foods. Their diet certainly contrasts with our North American fare of meat, potatoes, and processed food. The Japanese woman's lifestyle demonstrates that clearing up menopausal symptoms generally requires more than just a shift in attitude—but often less than a prescription for hormones. Over the years, many of my clients, the ones who have been unable to deal with hot flashes simply through minor lifestyle adjustments, have asked me if there is something they can take to alleviate this troublesome symptom. A vitamin or herb perhaps? Specific foods? The answer is yes. Making changes to your diet and your surroundings can definitely help you feel better. Below, I describe the natural approaches for treating hot flashes that I often recommend in my practice. Not only do my clients report improvement, but scientific studies also support the ability of these remedies to ease hot flashes.

dietary approaches

SOY FOODS AND ISOFLAVONES

Foods made from soybeans are certainly getting plenty of attention these days. (If you're wondering what these food are, you'll find a list on page 8). Scientists are learning that not only do soy foods have the ability to help protect us from heart disease, osteoporosis, and perhaps even cancer, but they can help ease menopausal hot flashes. A 12-week Italian study looked at the effects of soy protein on hot flashes in 104 women aged 48 to 61 years. The study found that, compared to the placebo group, the women who consumed 60 grams of soy protein powder daily reported a 26 percent reduction in the average number of hot flashes they experienced by their third week on this regimen, and a 33 percent reduction by the fourth week. At the end of the three-month study, the soy group had a 45 percent decrease in the number of hot flashes experienced daily. In comparison, the placebo group experienced only a 30 percent reduction.[1] Another study carried out by American researchers in North Carolina found that women whose daily diet included a total of 20 grams of soy protein reported significant improvement of hot flashes as well as of other menopausal symptoms.[2]

Now I don't want you to think that soy is the magic cure for hot flashes. It's true that a daily intake of soy has helped a number of my clients ease their hot flashes. But overall, studies don't find it to be a stupendously effective remedy. While it does tend to decrease both the frequency and severity of hot flashes, the effects are modest. And all the studies find that participating women who receive the placebo also experience some improvement. If a study finds that women who eat soy every day have 20 percent fewer hot flashes than women taking the dummy treatment, some experts might question the clinical relevance of the finding. Will a 20 percent improvement mean that much to your symptoms? Will it mean moving from 11 hot flashes per day down to 9? Don't get me wrong. I am a very big fan of soy foods, but I just don't want to overstate the effect soy has on hot flashes. On the other hand, I meet many women in my practice who tell me that any improvement is welcome.

You might be wondering what makes soybeans so special. Soybeans contain naturally occurring compounds called "isoflavones," which are a type of phytoestrogen (plant estrogen). Genistein and daidzein are the most active soy isoflavones and have been the focus of much research. Isoflavones have a molecular structure similar to that of the human estrogen hormones and as a result, have a weak estrogenic effect in the body. Even though soy isoflavones are about 50 times less potent than human estrogens, they are able to offer women a source of usable estrogen and, along with that, some of estrogen's protective effects. If a woman's estrogen levels are low enough to cause hot flashes during the perimenopausal or post-menopausal periods, a regular intake of foods like roasted soy nuts, soy beverages, and tofu may help to alleviate the situation. Foods like tofu and soy drinks can be eaten in delicious recipes and still be just as beneficial—the phytoestrogens in soy don't break down when heated.

How much should you eat?

Just how much soy you need has yet to be determined. You may have noticed that some experts recommend eating a certain amount of soy protein each day, while others specify an amount of phytoestrogens. Because soy foods can vary considerably with respect to their phytoestrogen content, I recommend getting a specific daily dose of phytoestrogens. Most studies that find soy foods helpful in treating hot flashes use enough of these foods to provide 65 milligrams of isoflavones daily. What's more, soy isoflavones seem to work best if they're taken twice per day. Depending on what type of soy food you eat, the isoflavone level in your bloodstream reaches a peak four to eight hours later. So it makes sense to get 30 milligrams of isoflavones two times daily to keep your blood levels up. Dr. Kenneth Setchell, a world-renowned expert on phytoestrogens at the University of Cincinnati College of Medicine and the Children's Hospital Medical Center in Cincinnati, believes that a daily intake of 50 to 90 milligrams of phytoestrogens is probably needed to help alleviate hot flashes and reduce other health risks associated with menopause and aging.

Here's a chart that will help you plan your soy food consumption so that you get at least 50 milligrams of phytoestrogens per day.

Soy Food	Serving Size	Isoflavone Content
Roasted soy nuts	1/4 cup (50 ml)	40–60 mg
Soybeans, cooked or canned	1/2 cup (125 ml)	14 mg
Tempeh, uncooked	4 oz. (120 g)	60 mg
Soy flour	1/4 cup (50 ml)	44 mg
Tofu, uncooked	4 oz. (120 g)	38 mg

Texturized vegetable protein, dry	1/2 cup (125 ml)	30–120 mg
Soy beverage, So Good brand™	1 cup (250 ml)	26 mg
Soy beverage, most brands	1 cup (250 ml)	25–60 mg
Soy sauce		none
Soya oil		none

Types of soy foods

The chart above might be more confusing than helpful if you're unfamiliar with soy foods. Here's a quick introduction to what these foods are, where you can get them, and how they're used in the kitchen.

Soybeans   You can buy these already cooked (in cans) or dried. Dried soybeans need to be soaked in water overnight before cooking. Add cooked soybeans to soups, casseroles, chilies, and curries, or mash them and add them to burgers. For a real treat, order *edemake* (green soybeans) as an appetizer in a Japanese restaurant.

Miso   A traditional Asian flavouring, miso is a paste made of a fermented mixture of soybeans and grain. Miso is excellent added to soups at the end of cooking, or in marinades and sauces. For vegetable soup, use one-quarter cup miso (50 millilitres) for every quart (or litre) of water.

Soy Flour   Soybeans can be defatted and finely ground to make a flour that is sold in health food stores and some grocery stores. Because soy flour contains no gluten, the wheat protein that adds structure to baked goods, it should be mixed with other flours in baking. Substitute soy flour for up to one-half of the wheat flour in breads, muffins, loaves, cakes, cookies, or scones.

Soy Beverages   These are made from either the juice of ground soybeans or from isolated soy protein. You'll find many different brands and flavours in grocery and health food stores. Try a few brands to find one with a taste you like—but be sure to buy a brand fortified with calcium and vitamin D. Use soy beverages just as you would milk—on cereal, and in smoothies, coffee, lattes, soups, and cooking and baking.

Soy "Meats"   These ready-to-eat or frozen soy foods resemble meat and can be used in place of burgers, hot dogs, deli cold cuts, and ground meat. You'll find them in the freezer, deli, or produce section of grocery stores. Remember that soy burgers and dogs are already cooked. Overcooking will dry them out and probably discourage you from trying them again. All they need is reheating on a hot grill.

Soy "Nuts"   Also called roasted soybeans, this snack food comes in plain, barbecue, and garlic flavours. Of all the soy foods, soy nuts have the highest amount of isoflavones per serving—two tablespoons pack roughly 42 milligrams! The good news for those of you who tend to like salty snack foods—these munchies have less salt, less fat, and more fibre than actual nuts, yet they're tasty and satisfying.

Tempeh   You'll find this traditional Asian soy food sold in small bars in the refrigerated or frozen food section of health food stores. Made of a fermented soybean-grain mixture, tempeh has a nutty, delicious flavour. Slice it and add it to casseroles and stir fries or grill it in kebabs and burgers. Tempeh is tastiest and most digestible when you simmer it in a marinade for 20 minutes before incorporating it into other recipes.

Texturized Vegetable Protein (TVP)   TVP is made from defatted and dehydrated soy flour. It's sold in packages of granules or small chunks. Rehydrate TVP with an equal amount of water or broth, then use it to replace ground meat in pasta sauces, lasagna, chili, and tacos.

Tofu   Tofu is made by using minerals or lemon juice to coagulate juice from soaked, ground, and briefly cooked soybeans. Tofu readily picks up flavours during cooking. It comes in soft (silken) or firm varieties. Use soft tofu in smoothies, dips, salad dressings, lasagna, and cheesecake recipes. Firm tofu is best for grilling and stir-frying—or add cubes of it to soups for a protein boost.

Cooking with soy foods

I can understand that if you've never tried soy foods before, you might feel hesitant about what to do with them. Tofu, especially, seems to have a bad reputation—many of my clients aren't used to eating soy foods and when I mention tofu I usually see noses turn up. You'd have thought I had just recommended eating Brussels sprouts. Then again, let's face it, a cake of soybean curd doesn't look that appealing and it's definitely a hard food to sneak into the family dinner. It might help to look at this as an opportunity to be adventurous. To assist you, I've prepared the following Nutrition Tip, "Ten Ways to Enjoy More Soy." If the tips don't help, try one of the recipes in Appendix 3. They all come highly recommended by my clients!

NUTRITION TIP

Ten ways to enjoy more soy

1 Use a fortified soy beverage on cereal or in a breakfast smoothie (see recipe in Appendix 3).

2 Use a fortified soy beverage in cooking and baking, for instance in soups, casseroles, muffins, and pancake batters.

3 Cube firm tofu and add to soups.

4 Grill firm tofu on the barbecue. First marinate tofu in balsamic vinegar or brush with hoisin sauce, then make tofu kebabs with vegetables.

5 Substitute soft or firm tofu for ricotta cheese in lasagna and cheesecake recipes.

6 Use silken tofu in creamy salad dressing or dip recipes.

7 Replace one-quarter of the all-purpose flour in a recipe with soy flour.

8 Snack on roasted soy nuts—they come in plain, barbecue, garlic, or onion flavours.

9 Replace ground meat with TVP (texturized vegetable protein) in chili, pasta sauce, and tacos.

10 Try veggie burgers (with soy protein) and veggie dogs cooked on the grill. When buying veggie burgers, make sure you see "soy protein" listed as one of the first few ingredients on the label.

Soy protein powders

If you've tried my recipe ideas and you're still not convinced that soy foods are welcome in your daily diet, consider using a high quality soy protein powder. It's easy to throw a scoop of soy protein powder into a homemade breakfast smoothie or a glass of orange juice. I have many clients who use these powders to ensure they get their daily dose of soy isoflavones.

Before you rush off to the health food store, however, keep in mind that soy protein powders vary in quality. Depending on how the manufacturer extracts the protein from the soybean, you can end up with a little or a lot of isoflavones. Look for products made with isolated soy protein. Soy protein isolates offer the purest form of soy protein available—the protein is completely separated, or isolated, from the carbohydrate and fat portions of the soybean. Most soy protein isolates are made using a water extraction process, which preserves the naturally occurring isoflavones. I don't recommend buying soy protein concentrates. Many of these are made using alcohol to extract the protein from the bean. Alcohol extraction causes a loss of naturally occurring isoflavones. If you're uncertain how the soy protein you're contemplating for purchase is made, call the manufacturer. Here's how the two protein extraction methods compare.

ISOFLAVONE CONTENT OF WATER- AND ALCOHOL-EXTRACTED SOY PROTEIN POWDERS

Type of Soy Protein	Serving Size	Isoflavone Content
Soy protein isolate (water extraction)	2 rounded tbsp. (30 g)	29.3 mg
Soy protein concentrate (water extraction)	2 rounded tbsp. (30 g)	30.6 mg
Soy protein concentrate (alcohol extraction)	2 rounded tbsp. (30 g)	3.7 mg

Source: USDA-Iowa State University Database on the Isoflavone Content of Foods 1999 Release 1.1

My advice is to buy a product made with Supro® brand soy protein. Manufactured by Protein Technologies International using an isoflavone-friendly process, Supro® soy protein isolate contains plenty of isoflavones. It's also the soy protein isolate used in scientific studies. Products that use Supro® include Genisoy Protein Powder, TWINLAB Vege Fuel®, GNC Challenge Soy Protein 95, GNC Challenge Soy Solution, Nutrel Soy Serenity and Soy Strategy, Naturade Total Soy, and Interactive SoyOne.

Isoflavone supplements

If you've been to your local health food store lately, you might have noticed a number of isoflavone supplements on the shelf. These supplements are made with isoflavones that have been extracted from soybeans or red clover plants. For many of you, I'm sure that popping an isoflavone pill with your multivitamin seems more appealing than eating a plate of stir-fried tofu. But the question is, do these supplements relieve hot flashes? Unfortunately, at the time of writing only a few completed studies exist that have tried to answer this question, and almost all have found these supplements to be ineffective.

One small study conducted at the Massachusetts Institute of Technology in Cambridge, Massachusetts, found no significant change in the number of hot flashes or night sweats experienced by postmenopausal women who took a soy isoflavone extract each day. Two Australian studies also found that isoflavone supplements had no effect on hot flashes. In one of these studies, 37 post-menopausal women were divided into three groups and given either placebo or 40 milligrams or 160 milligrams daily of isoflavone extract derived from red clovers (called Promensil™). In the second study, 51 post-menopausal women took 40 milligrams of Promensil™ daily (one tablet) for three months and reported no difference in menopausal symptoms.[3]

On a more positive note, a recent study presented at the 1999 Annual Meeting of the North American Menopause Society found that an isoflavone supplement made from soy helped alleviate hot flashes in post-menopausal women. A total of 177 women entered the trial. The average age of the trial participants was 55 and all were experiencing five or more hot flashes a day before the study. At the end of 12 weeks, women who had taken two 50-milligram isoflavone tablets daily experienced a significant reduction in severity of hot flashes compared to women who had been given the placebo. The researchers also found that that the supplement appeared to help reduce the number of hot flashes, but this finding wasn't statistically significant.[4]

Another preliminary study hailing from Tufts University in Boston asked 16 women to take Promensil™ every day for two to three months. After eight weeks on the supplement, study participants reported a significant decrease in the number and intensity of their hot flashes. While these results may sound encouraging, the researchers did not use a control group to compare the effects of Promensil™ to that of a placebo.[5]

So what should you do? Eat food or pop a pill? Most experts agree that for reasons not yet fully understood, soy isoflavones work best in combination with soy proteins. When it comes to reducing hot flashes, lowering cholesterol, or building bone mass, most studies have found isoflavone supplements alone to be ineffective. And because of the limited amount of research done on these products, we know little about their safety. Foods rich in soy protein contain isoflavones as well as many other protective compounds which appear to all work together to create the food's beneficial effects. Until scientists give the green light on isoflavone supplements, I recommend that you get your phytoestrogens from soy foods or soy protein isolate powders.

vitamins and minerals

VITAMIN E

If you're eating for a healthy heart, then chances are you're already familiar with this antioxidant vitamin (you'll read how vitamin E helps protect you from heart disease in Chapter 9). It seems that vitamin E might also help to reduce hot flashes. Unfortunately, very little research has been done on this subject, and much of it dates back to the late 1940s. Although these studies were not placebo controlled, they did find the vitamin to be effective in reducing hot flashes. I have managed to find one recent study from the Mayo Clinic and Mayo Foundation in Cleveland. During the first four weeks of the study, the researchers gave 120 women with a history of breast cancer 800 international units (IU) of vitamin E daily. After taking vitamin E for four weeks, the women were given an identical looking placebo pill. The women did report fewer hot flashes when taking vitamin E, but the effect was not dramatic. Despite the limited amount of research, a survey of 438 American women conducted by researchers at Columbia University in New York revealed that 57 percent who had hot flashes took vitamin E and 27 percent of these women felt that it helped.[6]

How the vitamin works to reduce hot flashes is not completely understood. Vitamin E has been reported to prevent excessive production of follicle stimulating hormone (FSH) and luteinizing hormone (LH). As discussed earlier in this chapter, the higher the levels of these two hormones in your body, the more your blood vessels dilate. This dilation, in turn, increases blood flow to the skin, causing you to feel hotter.

While there's not a lot of scientific support for vitamin E as a therapy for hot flash relief, I am in favour of adding it to your nutrition regime. As you'll read later in the book, vitamin E has other important health benefits and it's impossible to get high amounts in your daily diet. The richest sources of this vitamin are vegetable oils, nuts, seeds, and wheat germ. Leafy green vegetables like kale and collards are also good sources. But when you consider that one tablespoon of olive oil gives you a measly 2.6 IU of the vitamin, and two tablespoons of toasted wheat germ only give you 4 IU, you can see why you must rely on a supplement to get 400 or 800 IU.

BIOFLAVONOIDS AND VITAMIN C

Bioflavonoids are natural chemicals found in plant foods. They are especially plentiful in the inner peel of citrus fruits. They have been reported to have a very weak estrogen-like effect—they are about 50,000 times less potent than your body's own estrogen.

Over the years bioflavonoids have been used to treat hot flashes, as well as vaginal dryness and fluid retention. They're most often given together with vitamin C. It makes sense that the two work best together, since citrus fruits are rich sources of both. Despite the fact that I could not find any published clinical studies supporting their use for hot flash alleviation, bioflavonoids and vitamin C are worth a try. They're both relatively easy to get in the diet, and if taken in appropriate amounts in supplemental form, they pose no risk to otherwise healthy women.

To get more citrus bioflavonoids and vitamin C into your diet, aim to eat at least one citrus fruit, such as an orange or grapefruit, each day. Or drink a glass of unsweetened citrus juice. If you make your juice at home, you can also juice the fruit rinds. If you decide to try this, you may want to stick to unwaxed, organically grown fruits. And make sure to add freshly grated citrus peel to fruit salsas, green salads, salad dressings, and home baked muffins or loaves.

NUTRITION TIP

Boosting your C

Vitamin C is needed to synthesize collagen, a protein that provides support for blood vessel walls, scar tissue, and bones. Vitamin C also bolsters the body's immune system and strengthens resistance to infection. And it's needed to help the body absorb iron from whole grains, fruit, and vegetables. In fact, if you drink a glass of orange or grapefruit juice with your iron-fortified breakfast cereal, you'll absorb up to four times more of the iron.

Since the body can't store vitamin C, you have to consume enough every day through your diet. Health Canada's recommended daily intake for healthy adult women is 30 milligrams. If you're a smoker, however, you need to almost double this amount (aim to get 60 milligrams each day).

Getting enough vitamin C from your diet is relatively easy. For example, having one glass of orange juice at breakfast, a green salad at lunch, and a stalk of broccoli and baked potato with the skin at dinner will supply more than 300 milligrams of the vitamin. A one-half cup (125-millilitre) serving of raw or cooked broccoli, Brussels sprouts, or red pepper, or a one-half cup (125-millilitre) serving of cantaloupe or strawberries all provide more than 50 milligrams of vitamin C.

If you find it difficult to get adequate amounts of vitamin C and bioflavonoids from food, try a vitamin C supplement with added bioflavonoids (if bioflavonoids have been added, this will be stated on the label). Take a 500- to 600-milligram supplement once or twice daily—depending on the brand, one pill will give you approximately 50 to 100 milligrams of bioflavonoids. When you're choosing a vitamin C supplement, buy a product containing a special form of vitamin C known as "Ester-C®." This is a patented form of the vitamin that laboratory studies have found to be up to four times more available to the body than regular vitamin C (called ascorbic acid or ascorbate). Many supplement companies offer Ester-C®.

herbal remedies

BLACK COHOSH ROOT

Also known as squawroot, bugbane, and snakeroot, black cohosh (*Cimicifuga racemosa*) has long been used by North America's First Nations peoples for treating menstrual and menopausal symptoms. It's also popular in Europe, especially Germany. In Germany it's been used for over 40 years by more than 1.5 million women. Both my clinical experience with clients and the findings from controlled scientific studies indicate that black cohosh is definitely the most promising herbal remedy for treating menopausal symptoms.

When it comes to relieving hot flashes, many studies have found black cohosh to be just as effective as estrogen therapy. How the herb works, though, is currently under scientific debate—in other words, we're not really sure!

Experts do agree that naturally occurring active compounds in black cohosh are able to lower levels of luteinizing hormone (LH)—as you'll recall, high LH levels can trigger hot flashes. These active compounds are called triterpene glycosides or more generally, phytoestrogens, and are thus in the same class of compounds as the isoflavones found in soybeans. Where the experts don't agree is how these triterpene glycosides actually lower LH levels. Many German studies seem to indicate that they work by acting like weak estrogen molecules and binding to estrogen receptors. However, recent research has demonstrated that the herb does not have an estrogenic effect and instead, it may lower blood levels of LH by acting on receptors in the brain (remember, it's the hypothalamus that tells your pituitary gland to make LH).[7] Regardless of how black cohosh works to ease hot flashes, its effectiveness has helped many women through menopause.

The advantage black cohosh offers in treating hot flashes is that it doesn't have the side effects associated with hormone therapy. Black cohosh should be your first treatment of choice if estrogen therapy is not an option because of uncomfortable side effects or because you have a higher risk of developing breast cancer. Of course, those of you who have had estrogen-positive breast cancer will likely have an important question to pose here. If black cohosh acts like estrogen, will it increase your risk of getting breast cancer again? The answer is no. A recent study found that black cohosh does not cause estrogen-positive breast cancer cells to grow. Furthermore, the researchers showed that the herb was able to inhibit, rather than promote, the growth of cancer cells.[8] The only side effect that's been reported in a small number of women is mild stomach upset.

RESEARCH FILE

Black cohosh and hot flashes

Need some scientific evidence to help you decide whether or not you'll try an herbal remedy? I certainly don't blame you. In fact, I always make sure that carefully designed scientific research has been done that demonstrates the effectiveness of any herbal remedy I recommend to clients (that goes for vitamins and foods too!). When it comes to black cohosh, the research is not lacking, and positive results have emerged from well controlled studies. At the time of writing this book, eight clinical studies have been reported. Here's a look at a few of the findings:

- **1987, Germany**   In this randomized trial, 80 perimenopausal women were given black cohosh root (Remifemin™), standard estrogen therapy, or placebo. After 12 weeks, only the black cohosh extract had significantly improved hot flashes (as well as vaginal dryness and mood changes).

- **1988, Germany**   This study followed 60 women under 40 years of age who had had a hysterectomy. Women were randomly assigned either one of three estrogen medications or a standardized extract of black cohosh root (Remifemin™). After six months, all groups had experienced a significant decline in menopausal symptoms. In this study, the herb was just as effective as estrogen in reducing hot flashes.
- **1991, Germany**   Researchers compared black cohosh to placebo with respect to its ability to affect hormone levels in 110 women with menopausal symptoms. After six months, there was a significant drop in the levels of luteinizing hormone (LH) in the black cohosh group. (Remember, the higher your LH levels, the more your blood vessels dilate, increasing blood flow to the skin and making you feel hotter.) Again, Remifemin™ extract was used.[9]

As stated above, I often recommend buying the herbal product used in the scientific research, which in the case of black cohosh, is Remifemin™. This product in available in supplement stores, health food stores, and some pharmacies. There are also many other brands that use top quality ingredients and make an effective product. Here's a rule to follow when buying almost any herbal remedy: always buy a product standardized to contain a specified amount of the herb's active ingredient. When an herbal remedy has been standardized, each pill or capsule is guaranteed to give you a the specified amount of the active ingredient responsible for the herb's effects. By choosing a standardized product, you're making sure you get your money's worth. Unstandardized brands could contain little, or no, active ingredients. With black cohosh, you're looking for the words "triterpene glycosides." High quality brands state on the label that each tablet or capsule provides 40 milligrams of black cohosh standardized to contain 2.5 percent triterpene glycosides.

While Remifemin™ is sold in 20-milligram tablets, most other brands of black cohosh are sold in 40-milligram tablets. This is because almost all of the studies done with menopausal women used either 40 milligrams twice daily or double this amount, 80 milligrams twice daily. I recommend that you start with 40 milligrams twice a day. Improvement is usually noticed four to eight weeks after you start taking the herb. If you don't notice any change in your hot flashes after six weeks, increase your dosage to 80 milligrams twice daily, but keep in mind that as you increase your dose, you may experience mild stomach upset.

THE bottom LINE...

Leslie's recommendations for relieving hot flashes

1   Eliminate from your diet foods that can make hot flashes worse. Foods and beverages that contain caffeine are prime culprits. Keep your alcohol intake down to no more than one drink per day. Avoid alcohol altogether if you're experiencing hot flashes or if you're under stress. Finally, stay away from spicy foods.

2   Add one serving of soy food to your diet each day.

3   Ensure you're eating 50 milligrams of isoflavones each day.

4   If you're having trouble eating enough soy foods to give you 50 milligrams of isoflavones daily, add 1 to 2 tablespoons (15 to 25 millilitres) of a soy protein powder (made from soy protein isolate) to milk, juice, or a homemade fruit smoothie daily.

5   Start taking 400 IU of vitamin E each day and increase your dosage to 800 IU if necessary. Buy natural source vitamin E. Vitamin E is fat soluble, so take it with a meal that contains a little fat to help its absorption. Don't take vitamin E if you're on blood thinning medication. Check with your physician first.

6   To get more bioflavonoids and vitamin C, add one citrus fruit to your diet each day. Add citrus zest to recipes where appropriate.

7   Take a 500- or 600-milligram supplement of Ester-C® (a special form of vitamin C) with added bioflavonoids once or twice daily. Or, buy a separate bioflavonaid suppliement of 250 to 500 milligrams.

8   If you've done all this and your hot flashes are still bothersome, take a standardized extract of black cohosh root. Start with 40 milligrams of the herb, twice daily, morning and evening (40 milligrams is usually the amount found in one tablet or capsule). If you don't find the herb effective after six weeks, take two 40-milligram tablets twice daily.

restless nights and insomnia

"I started waking up to find my body soaking wet and cold and the bed sheets literally drenched. I found myself in a constant state of exhaustion. I had to find a cure for these night sweats if I was going to be able to perform properly during the workday."

2

How many of you have woken up feeling hot and bothered, your bed sheets soaking wet? Night sweats cause disrupted sleep in a good number of women in their peri- and post-menopausal years. While many women have no difficulty falling back to sleep, some simply cannot. Night after night of little sleep leaves them feeling exhausted, and that's when many other menopausal symptoms can emerge. Fatigue can lead to irritability, depression, and forgetfulness. But don't get me wrong—I'm not saying that insomnia is the only reason for these symptoms. Hormonal fluctuations that accompany the perimenopausal years can be responsible too. You'll learn more about these fluctuations and their overall potential impact in Chapters 3 and 4.

While insomnia may be the result of nocturnal hot flashes in some cases, some experts believe that something else, something unrelated to hot flashes, interrupts sleep in many peri- and post-menopausal women. Whatever is causing your sleepless nights, you can take action without resorting to prescribed sleeping aids (or a belt of scotch!) before tucking in for the night.

dietary approaches

CUT DOWN ON THE CAFFEINE

No doubt you've heard this before—eat and drink fewer caffeine-containing foods and beverages and you'll sleep better. Still, it's advice that bears repeating. Caffeine stimulates the central nervous system. While one or two cups of coffee in the morning may give you that gentle lift you were hoping for, the fourth or fifth cup can overstimulate your system and cause insomnia (not to mention irritability). My first recommendation to clients wanting to cut down is to avoid caffeine in the afternoon. Replace caffeine-containing beverages with caffeine-free or decaffeinated beverages like herbal tea, mineral water, unsweetened fruit or vegetable juice, or decaffeinated coffee.

How much caffeine is too much?

Health Canada says that a daily consumption of 400 to 450 milligrams of caffeine does not pose any risks for healthy people.[1] But remember, Health Canada's recommendation is based on studies that have investigated the effect of caffeine on blood pressure and other health conditions, not on your ability to sleep soundly. While Health Canada's upper limit of 450 milligrams won't harm your health, it may keep you up at night—and that may harm your health! Studies have shown that as little as one or two cups of coffee in the morning will affect the quality of your sleep that night. Other studies have found that as little as 100 milligrams of caffeine (the amount found in four ounces or 125 millilitres of coffee) can delay sleep when taken before bedtime, especially in people who don't normally consume caffeine.[2] Caffeine blocks the action of adenosine, a natural brain chemical that slows the body down. If you're having trouble getting to sleep, or you're waking up during the night, aim to consume no more than 200 milligrams per day, and preferably much less.

NUTRITION TIP

Minding your caffeine

Use this chart to find out how much caffeine you're consuming. (And remember that the "Grande" sized cup at Starbucks contains a lot more than six ounces!)

CAFFEINE CONTENT OF COMMON FOODS AND BEVERAGES (MILLIGRAMS)

Coffee, filter drip, 6 oz. (187 ml)	110–180
Coffee, instant, 6 oz. (187 ml)	60–90
Espresso, 2 oz. (60 ml)	90–100
Tea, black, 6 oz. (187 ml)	35
Tea, green, 6 oz. (187 ml)	25
Cola, 12 oz. (375 ml)	35
Dark chocolate, 2 oz. (60 g)	40–50
Chocolate cake, 1 slice	20–30
Excedrin®, 2 tablets	130
Anacin® or Midol, 2 tablets	64

ELIMINATE ALCOHOL

Unfortunately, there are no two ways about it—the effects of alcohol are detrimental to sleep and consuming alcohol will worsen insomnia. Even if you're not suffering from sleep problems, a few drinks certainly can affect the quality of your sleep. Swiss researchers have found that taking a moderate amount of alcohol six hours before bedtime reduces sleep time and increases wakefulness twofold. I know that if I enjoy a couple of glasses of wine in the evening, I inevitably wake up a few times that night. Or worse, I wake up at four in the morning, and can't get back to sleep. Then I'm forced to drag myself through the next day feeling tired and lethargic. Sound familiar? I can remember the good old days when a few drinks wouldn't bother me—I could stay out late and feel great on less than eight hours of sleep. Well, being the good nutritionist I am, I now save my alcohol for the weekend when I can grab a few extra hours of sleep each night. For the sake of sound sleep, a healthy body, and a productive mind, I recommend the same to all my clients.

Do you ever wonder why alcohol affects sleep the way it does? Once absorbed into the bloodstream, alcohol is metabolized (or processed) by the liver at a set rate. If you drink more alcohol than your liver can keep up with (about one drink per hour), alcohol arrives in the brain where it interferes with brain chemicals called neurotransmitters, which are responsible for the transfer of messages from one nerve cell to another.

The neurotransmitters need to be in proper balance for deep, restful sleep to occur. Alcohol has also been reported to impair the REM portion of sleep, a sleep phase very important for physical, emotional, and mental restoration.[3]

At the same time that alcohol robs you of rest, it also tires you further by dehydrating you. Alcohol's dehydrating effect is due to its ability to depress the brain's production of antidiuretic hormone. Without enough antidiuretic hormone, you lose water and minerals through the kidneys. This, in turn, can increase your feeling of fatigue. That's because water makes it possible for you to digest, absorb, and transport nutrients throughout your body. So when you're dehydrated after an evening of drinking alcohol, your cells receive nutrients less efficiently. You also need water to help regulate your body temperature. If you drink too much alcohol (even just a couple of drinks) your body will have trouble properly regulating its temperature. If you're well hydrated, your body has enough fluid to release heat that builds up due to normal metabolism and exercise—every day your body releases heat through your skin in the form of sweat. If you're dehydrated because you're not drinking enough fluids, or you've enjoyed a little too much wine, your body can't release built up heat as efficiently because it doesn't have enough fluid to produce sweat. As a result, you may find your hot flashes get worse after imbibing.

How much alcohol is safe?

If we're talking about health protection, I recommend no more than seven drinks per week for women. This recommendation is based on our current knowledge regarding cancer prevention. But if you're suffering from insomnia, or you want to be at your peak the next day, I suggest you eliminate alcohol from your diet. Instead of having a glass of wine, pour yourself sparkling mineral water and spruce it up with a slice of lime. Or try some of the non-alcoholic wines or beers available. If you're looking for a cocktail, I suggest a virgin Caesar, tomato juice, or a splash of cranberry juice in soda water.

You can also use a few tricks to lessen the effect of alcohol on your sleep:

Drink alcohol with a meal or snack. If you drink alcohol on an empty stomach, about 20 percent is absorbed directly across the walls of your stomach and reaches the brain within a minute. But when the stomach is full of food, alcohol has less chance of touching its walls and passing through them, so the effect on your brain is delayed.

Drink no more than one drink every hour. Since the liver can't metabolize alcohol any faster than this, drinking slowly will ensure your blood alcohol concentration doesn't rise. To help you slow your pace, try alternating alcoholic and non-alcoholic drinks. By the way, one drink is equivalent to 5 ounces (150 millilitres) of wine, 12 ounces (375 millilitres) of beer, 10 ounces (310 millilitres) of wine cooler, or 1.5 ounces (45 millilitres) of liquor. A pint of beer (500 millilitres) counts as two drinks!

EAT CARBOHYDRATE BEFORE BED

If your mother ever told you to drink a glass of warm glass of milk to help you sleep, she was smart. A snack rich in carbohydrate, like a glass of milk, a small bowl of cereal, or a slice of toast, provides the brain with an amino acid called tryptophan. The brain needs tryptophan to manufacture a neurotransmitter called serotonin. And serotonin has been shown to facilitate sleep, improve mood, diminish pain, and even reduce appetite.

I don't often recommend snacks after dinner, especially for clients who are trying to lose weight. But if you follow this suggestion in the spirit I've intended, you won't gain weight. If you want to find out whether carbohydrate helps you fall asleep, eat a small amount of carbohydrate food, or drink a glass of low fat milk or soy beverage one hour before going to bed. Try this strategy for a week. If your insomnia does not improve, look at other factors that may be disrupting your sleep.

vitamins and minerals

VITAMIN B12

Many studies have found that vitamin B12 promotes sleep, especially in people with sleep disorders. Researchers in Japan have used 1.5 to 3 milligrams of the vitamin each day to restore normal sleep patterns in patients. When vitamin B12 was withheld for two months, sleep disruptions reappeared. A German study found that sleep quality, ability to concentrate, and "feeling refreshed" were significantly correlated with B12 blood levels in healthy men and women.[4]

Exactly how this B vitamin works to influence sleep is not completely understood. Some researchers believe it interacts with melatonin, a natural hormone in the body. Melatonin is involved in maintaining the body's internal clock, which, in turn, regulates the secretion of various hormones. In so doing, melatonin is also thought to help control sleep and wakefulness patterns. Melatonin production is stimulated by darkness and suppressed by light. It seems that vitamin B12 directly influences melatonin release and metabolism and may prevent disturbances in melatonin balance.

The established recommended dietary allowance (RDA) of vitamin B12 for healthy adults (women and men) is 2.4 micrograms per day. In 1998, the Food and Nutrition Board of the National Academy of Sciences, an organization of American and Canadian scientists who set RDAs for North America, made a new recommendation regarding vitamin B12, saying that people over the age of 50 should get their B12 by eating foods fortified with the vitamin, or by taking a supplement. The board made this recommendation because it is known that up to 30 percent of older adults have lost the ability to properly absorb naturally occurring B12 in foods. To absorb vitamin B12, we must first separate it from food molecules with stomach acid. As we get older, we start to produce less stomach acid. It's estimated that 30 percent of older adults produce very little, or no acid, a condition called achlorhydria.

What about a vitamin B12 supplement?

Vitamin B12 is found in all animal foods—meat, poultry, fish, eggs, and dairy products. If you are eating these foods every day, chances are you are meeting your need for B12. Foods fortified with the vitamin include soy beverages, rice beverages, and breakfast cereals (you'll have to check the label to be sure). If you fall into one of the following categories, however, I do recommend you take a B12 supplement:

- You're over 50 years of age.
- You're taking antacid medication for reflux (heartburn) or a stomach ulcer.
- You're a strict vegetarian who eats no animal foods.

Vitamin B12 supplements come in 500 or 1,000 microgram sizes. To ensure you're meeting your requirements, I recommend 500 micrograms once a day, with a meal. The active form of vitamin B12, called methylcobalamin, is preferred over cyanocobalamin.

NUTRITION TIP

Boosting your B12

Nutrition authorities agree that you need 2.4 micrograms of vitamin B12 each day. Are you getting enough? Well, here's a list of foods high in B12 that will help you boost your intake in no time.

VITAMIN B12 CONTENT OF COMMON FOODS (MICROGRAMS)

Beef, flank, cooked, 3 oz. (90 g)	2.8
Pork centre loin, cooked, 3 oz. (90 g)	0.5
Chicken breast, cooked, 5 oz. (140 g)	0.3
Chicken leg, cooked, 6 oz. (180 g)	0.2
Salmon, sockeye, cooked, 3 oz. (90 g)	4.9
Tuna, canned and drained, 3 oz. (90 g)	2.5
Mussels, cooked, 3 oz. (90 g)	20
Milk, 1 cup (250 ml)	0.9
Yogurt, 3/4 cup (175 ml)	0.9
Cheese, cheddar 1 oz. (30 g)	0.2
Cottage cheese, 1%, 1/2 cup (125 ml)	0.7
Egg, 1 whole	0.6
Fortified soy drink, 1 cup (250 ml)	1.0
Fortified rice drink, 1 cup (250 ml)	1.0

herbal remedies

VALERIAN

Native to Europe, this plant has a mild sedative effect on the central nervous system. Valerian root (*Valeriana officinalis*) makes getting to sleep easier and it increases the amount of time you spend in deep sleep. Unlike popular prescribed sleeping pills, valerian does not lead to dependence or addiction. And it usually doesn't cause a morning "hangover"—when compared to drugs like Valium® and Xanax®, valerian binds very weakly to brain receptors.[5] Scientists have learned that valerian promotes sleep by increasing the levels of a brain chemical called gamma-aminobutyric acid (GABA).

GABA plays a key role in reducing feelings of stress and anxiety. Scientists can actually measure an increased concentration of GABA in the brains of individuals who have taken valerian. And, it seems, not only is valerian able to increase the amount of GABA the brain secretes, it also helps prevent the levels from falling too quickly. The net result for someone who takes valerian is that GABA levels stay high for a longer period of time.

Much of the research on valerian and sleep dates back to the mid-1980s and early 1990s. At least 10 controlled clinical studies have evaluated valerian's effects in both healthy people and in patients with sleep disorders. In one double blind study (both the researchers and the subjects didn't know who was getting valerian or placebo), 89 percent of those taking 400 milligrams of valerian root reported improved sleep; indeed 44 percent of the study participants taking valerian reported perfect sleep. Two other studies done with healthy people found that valerian was able to significantly reduce the time it takes to fall asleep and improve the quality of sleep. In both studies, participants used 400 to 450 milligrams of valerian daily.

Although the active ingredients in valerian have not yet been confirmed, many experts attribute the herb's effect to certain essential oils found in the root. For this reason, I recommend that you buy a product standardized to contain at least 0.5 percent essential oils or 0.8 percent valerenic acid. Take 400 to 600 milligrams in capsule or tablet form, from 45 minutes to one hour before going to bed. If you wake up feeling groggy, reduce the dose. And don't expect results overnight. One German study found that the herb worked better for people suffering chronic insomnia when used over a period of time.[6] Valerian has a delayed onset of action and it should be taken for two to four weeks to achieve an improvement in sleep.

No side effects or contraindications are known. The German Commission E reports that valerian is safe to use during pregnancy and breast-feeding. (In case you're wondering what the Commission E is, it's a body established by the German government to evaluate the safety and efficacy of herbs available for general use. Information on herbal remedies from Commission E is considered the most accurate available.)

other ways to help yourself sleep

Here are some further suggestions for increasing your likelihood of getting a restful night's sleep:

1   Don't forget about exercise. Regular physical activity can bring on a feeling of tiredness later in the day. And research shows exercise also helps you rest better by increasing your blood level of melatonin, which, as I discussed above, plays an important role in regulating sleep-wake cycles. I recommend a minimum of three to four cardiovascular exercise sessions each week. Try brisk walking, jogging, biking, stair climbing, swimming, cross-country skiing, or aerobics classes. If you haven't been exercising at all, see your doctor before you begin. Then start at 20 minutes per session and gradually build up to 30 to 45 minutes each time. Avoid exercising too close to bedtime (in other words, after dinner) since vigorous activity before going to bed may keep you awake a little longer.

2   Get into a nighttime routine that you associate with going to sleep. Reading a book, drinking a cup of chamomile tea, or taking a warm bath can all help slow your mind and body, preparing you for sleep. Avoid watching television or doing office work within one hour before your bedtime. Instead, do something that helps you quiet your mind and relax.

3   If worries and tension related to stress are keeping you awake at night, practise relaxation techniques. Learn about deep breathing or meditation. I have many clients who practise yoga regularly and can't say enough about its relaxing effect. If these techniques don't work for you, consider speaking with a stress management counselor.

4   When you've done everything right and you still can't sleep (or you have no energy) it's time to visit your family doctor. Both poor sleep patterns and ongoing fatigue may be the symptoms of an underlying health problem. A physical exam and blood tests can often help determine the cause.

    • Sleep disturbances can cause a loss of restorative sleep, the period during which your body rebuilds its vital forces. Depression, stress, obesity, muscle cramps, restless legs, and sleep-related breathing disorders such as sleep apnea can all interfere with a good night's rest. Referral to a sleep disorder clinic may be appropriate to determine the underlying cause of ongoing sleep disturbances.

THE Bottom LINE...

Leslie's recommendations for coping with insomnia

1   Cut back your caffeine intake to a daily maximum of 450 milligrams. Preferably, however, consume less than 200 milligrams daily.

2   If you do drink alcohol and you don't want to give it up (which I recommend doing if you're experiencing sleep problems), aim for no more than seven drinks per week. To lessen alcohol's impact on your brain, have your drink with a meal or a snack.

3   Try a light carbohydrate-rich snack 30 to 60 minutes before going to bed to increase the level of sleep-promoting serotonin in your brain. Good choices include a banana, a slice of toast, a glass of milk or calcium-fortified soy beverage, or a small bowl of cereal.

4   Make sure you get enough B12 in your diet. If you can't get enough B12 through food, or if you don't produce enough stomach acid to absorb it efficiently, take 500 micrograms of vitamin B12 in supplement form daily.

5   For short-term insomnia, consider taking 400 to 600 milligrams of valerian root extract one to two hours before going to bed. Buy a product standardized to contain at least 0.5 percent essential oils or 0.8 percent valerenic acid. Use valerian to manage acute bouts of insomnia. Long-term (longer than three months) daily use of valerian may cause headaches and sleepiness in some individuals.

6   Don't forget to investigate other possible causes of chronic sleep problems: a lack of exercise, too much stress, or a possible medical problem.

mood swings

"One minute I feel fine; the next minute I am irritable, cranky, irrational, and depressed for no particular reason. I am normally a high energy type person, but I find that I just can't get myself in gear these days, no matter how well I eat, sleep, or exercise."

3

Most women describe the mood swings of perimenopause as being like those of premenstrual syndrome (PMS). They talk about crying at the drop of a hat, or blowing up at a family member for no good reason. Some women describe day-long bad moods when everyone and everything annoys them. If you've ever suffered through these kinds of feelings during the premenstrual period, then you know they're not fun. And they can be disruptive to your personal and work life.

Not all women experience mood swings during the transition years, however. Studies show that if a woman has had a hysterectomy she's more likely to become depressed.[1] And it's my clinical observation that women who tend to be irritable and cranky during the premenstrual period experience the same mood swings at perimenopause. Those mood changes may be minor for some women and major for others.

Mood swings are partly due to a loss of estrogen. Although we don't yet fully understand what happens in the body during a woman's menstrual cycle, we do know that natural chemicals in the brain, called neurotransmitters, respond to hormonal fluctuations that occur during the cycle. Neurotransmitters are responsible for the transfer of messages from one nerve cell to another. These chemicals are released at the end of a nerve cell when a nerve impulse arrives there. Once they are released, neurotransmitters move to the next nerve cell and alter the membrane of that second cell so as to either inhibit or excite it. The neurotransmitters that excite nerve fibres make us more alert, while the ones that inhibit nerve fibres calm us down.

The hormonal ups and downs of perimenopause may also make us more sensitive than usual to our feelings. And certainly for some women the approach of menopause itself can be upsetting. If you're unhappy or dissatisfied with your life, the signal that one life phase is ending and a new one is beginning can be quite distressing. Sometimes a feeling of unfulfillment, whether it's a result of boredom at work or of an unhappy marriage, can create anxiety about the post-menopausal years—we fear that if we're not happy now, menopause will make matters worse. Other women fear they are leaving behind their youthful, productive years.

Regardless of what is responsible for your mood swings, there are things you can do to calm them down. Especially if they're interfering with your enjoyment of life, it's important to take action. If my suggestions don't help and your mood changes continue to disrupt your life, consult your family doctor.

dietary approaches

For centuries, people have used food to alter their mood. What our ancestors didn't realize was that by eating certain foods they were actually influencing their brain chemistry. Modern science, however, now recognizes that the foods we eat can affect our mood by modifying the brain's production and release of neurotransmitters. Our brain and nervous system rely on thirty to forty neurotransmitters to do their work; researchers believe that five or six of these can be affected by food. Nutrients like carbohydrates, proteins, and vitamins are able to cross the "blood-brain barrier"—a physiological mechanism that limits the types of substances that can enter the brain—and be converted into neurotransmitters.

Studies have shown that specific neurotransmitters affect our mood in predictable ways. It's not known for sure, though, whether eating meals designed to increase the level of certain neurotransmitters is an effective way to recreate the moods inspired by that neurotransmitter. Keep in mind that everyone is different and we may not all respond in the same way. What is true, however, is that any drastic change in your normal eating patterns (crash dieting, binging on sweets, or skipping meals) can alter neurotransmitter levels and your mood. So the first step to smoothing out your mood is to eat at regular intervals throughout the day—don't wait more than four to five hours between meals, and if you do have to go longer than that without eating, grab a between-meal snack. No more meal skipping! The second step? Eliminate caffeine and alcohol, two beverages known to increase anxiety, irritability, and feelings of depression. Your next step? Read on!

CARBOHYDRATE-RICH FOODS

Without a doubt, carbohydrates have been one of the most widely studied nutrients with respect to their effect on mood. High carbohydrate meals have been associated with a calming, relaxing effect and even drowsiness. A high carbohydrate meal like pasta increases the brain levels of an amino acid called tryptophan. The brain then uses tryptophan to make the neurotransmitter serotonin. Many studies have linked high serotonin levels with happier moods and low levels with mild depression and irritability. Most of the research in this area has been done with women who have PMS. One study found that meals high in carbohydrate improved mood in young women within 30 minutes of consumption. Another study found that when women with PMS took a high carbohydrate drink their mood improved within 90 minutes.[2]

If you're feeling depressed or irritable, try a high carbohydrate meal that contains very little protein. Since protein foods are made up of many different amino acids, the more protein you eat, whether it's chicken, meat, or fish, the more amino acids will enter your bloodstream. And that means there will be many other amino acids available to compete with tryptophan for entry into the brain. Remember that you want tryptophan levels to rise in your brain so that you can produce more serotonin, which can make you feel calm and relaxed. Try pasta with tomato sauce, a toasted whole grain bagel with jam, or a bowl of cereal with low fat milk.

If your mood needs a boost during the day, reach for a high carbohydrate beverage. In fact, the next time you're in the United States, drop by a pharmacy and pick up a liquid dietary supplement called PMS Escape. It's a powdered drink mix that comes in several flavours made from a blend of carbohydrates, vitamins, and minerals. It's thought to act by boosting serotonin levels in the brain. The product was developed by Judith Wurtman, Ph.D, a research scientist at the Massachusetts Institute of Technology (MIT) and a pioneer researcher of the carbohydrate-serotonin connection.

If your next vacation or business trip doesn't take you across the border, buy a carbohydrate replacement drink from your local health food store or sports equipment store. These drinks are used by athletes to help rebuild muscle carbohydrate stores after a hard workout. They're sold as powder mixes or ready-to-drink and come in a variety of flavours.

RESEARCH FILE

Attention chocoholics!

Ever wondered why chocolate lifts your spirits? Well, it seems there just might be a scientific explanation. Researchers attribute chocolate's mood enhancing ability to a number of its ingredients.

- The sugar in chocolate triggers the release of serotonin in the brain, producing a calm, relaxed feeling. Interestingly though, one recent study looked at chocolate addicts and found that after eating chocolate, mood did not improve. In fact, these women felt guilty after eating chocolate. The researchers summarized: "Although chocolate is a food which provides pleasure, for those who consider themselves chocolate addicts, any pleasure experienced is short lived and accompanied by feelings of guilt."
- The caffeine in chocolate stimulates the central nervous system to give you a quick lift. Since milk chocolate contains very little caffeine, dark chocolate is more likely to give you a hit.
- Chocolate contains fat-like compounds that have been shown to target receptors in the brain and produce heightened sensitivity and euphoria.[3]

Other experts argue that our love of chocolate is purely sensory, and that it's our desire for chocolate's wonderful smell, flavour, and rich texture that keeps us coming back for more (sounds about right to me). Indeed, at this time, most of the evidence linking chocolate with mood improvement is anecdotal. Still, it's nice to be able to justify that (occasional) chocolate bar!

OMEGA-3 FATS

It seems that the type of fat you eat can affect your mood. Scientists have learned that levels of omega-3 fats are lower in people who are depressed.[4] These special polyunsaturated oils are important components of nerve and brain cell membranes and help cells communicate messages effectively. Omega-3 fats may also be crucial for the formation of brain hormones that help stabilize mood.

The best sources of omega-3 oils are cold water fish. Salmon, mackerel, herring, sardines, and fresh tuna are good choices. They all contain two special omega-3 fats with long, barely pronounceable names: docosahexaenoic acid (DHA) and eicosapentaenoic acid (EPA). It's a lack of DHA that seems to be an important factor in depression. If you don't care to eat fish, there are other ways to get more DHA into your cell membranes. You body uses foods rich in a fat called alpha-linolenic acid to make DHA. Flaxseed oil, canola oil, walnut oil, soybeans, and green leafy vegetables all contain alpha-linolenic acid, an essential fatty acid that must be supplied in the diet. If you don't get enough of this fatty acid, your body can't make DHA. With today's emphasis on low fat and fat free products, many experts fear we're not getting enough alpha-linolenic acid.

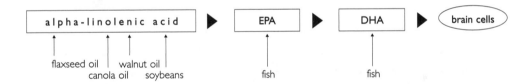

You'll see later on that the omega-3 family of fats does more than just prevent depression. Studies show that these fats appear to play important roles in fighting heart disease and breast cancer. But more on that later. In the meantime, concentrate on getting more omega-3 fats into your diet. Try to eat fish at least three times per week. Omega-3 eggs are another way to get more alpha-linolenic acid into your diet. The chickens that lay these eggs eat a diet high in flaxseed! One egg provides about 25 to 33 percent of the recommended daily intake of omega-3 fatty acids. Use flaxseed oil in salad dressings and canola oil in baking and cooking. In fact, try to get the majority of your added fats and oils from omega-3 sources. If you're allowing yourself four teaspoons (20 millilitres) of added fat a day, make sure that two or three of these (10 to 15 millilitres) come from omega-3 sources.

RESEARCH FILE

Fish oils and depression

Many studies have suggested that a lack of omega-3 fats in a person's diet is an important factor in depression. Scientists have found that the omega-3 content of red blood cell membranes is lower in people who are depressed. Does that mean that if you eat more omega-3 fats, like fish oil, your depression will lift? Well, Boston researchers from Harvard University and the Brigham and Women's Hospital have tried to answer that question. They studied 30 individuals with manic depression (also known as bipolar disorder) who were taking medication. The four-month study found that compared to placebo pills, people taking a daily dose of omega-3s from fish oil capsules had significantly longer remission periods from their depression. In fact, those who took the fish oil were three times more likely to maintain stable moods.[5]

While this research is interesting, it doesn't mean you should rush out to buy fish oil capsules if you're feeling a little down. Keep in mind that this was a study involving people with serious depression, serious enough to put them on medication. And fish oil supplements can be dangerous if taken in large doses for a long period of time. They contain a fair amount of vitamins A and D, which can be toxic in large doses. Your best bet is to follow my recommendations for getting enough omega-3 fat into your daily diet. And if you don't like eating fish and want to add a supplement, speak to your nutritionist or physician first.

Using flax oil

If you've never used flaxseed oil before you might like a few pointers. First of all, you won't find this healthy oil in your local supermarket. You'll have to make a trip to a health food store where you'll find it in the refrigerated foods section. Make sure you buy a brand bottled in opaque plastic or dark glass. And when you take the flaxseed oil home, put it right back in your fridge—omega-3 fats are sensitive to light and heat and turn rancid quickly if not stored properly. Because of its sensitivity to heat, flaxseed oil should never be used in recipes that call for heating. Instead, use this oil in salad dressings, dips, and other unheated dishes. If you want to add it to a cooked dish like soup, do so just before serving. Check out www.omeganutrition.com for recipes using flaxseed oil.

vitamins and minerals

VITAMIN B6

Even marginal deficiencies of the B vitamins have been associated with irritability, depression, and mood changes. For instance, one study found that vitamin B6-deficient mothers were less responsive to their newborns and were more likely to have older siblings care for them than mothers who consumed adequate amounts of B6. If you have ever suffered from PMS, chances are that you have already heard about vitamin B6. This B vitamin has been the focus of study in more than 900 women suffering from PMS (nine clinical studies have been published at the time of this writing). A recent review of this research found that doses of vitamin B6 of up to 100 milligrams daily bring about significant improvement in premenstrual symptoms.[6] Based on the evidence available, and the relationship I've observed between the mood swings of PMS and perimenopause, a daily supplement of vitamin B6 seems likely to improve your mood and smooth out the emotional roller coaster rides experienced by women suffering from perimenopausal depression or mood swings.

How does this vitamin affect your mood? Well, we find ourselves returning to that soothing brain chemical, serotonin. It turns out that the body uses vitamin B6 to form an important enzyme needed to convert the amino acid tryptophan into serotonin in the brain.

Healthy women need 1.6 milligrams of vitamin B6 each day. The best sources of B6 are high protein foods like meat, fish, and poultry. Other good sources include whole grains, bananas, and potatoes.

NUTRITION TIP
Boosting your B6
If your diet lacks protein foods and whole grains, chances are you're running low on vitamin B6. Here are a few foods that will pack more B6 into your diet.

VITAMIN B6 CONTENT OF COMMON FOODS (MILLIGRAMS)
Meat

Beef, flank, cooked, 3 oz. (90 g)	0.3
Pork centre loin, cooked, 3 oz. (90 g)	0.3

Chicken breast, cooked, 4.5 oz. (140 g)	0.3
Chicken leg, cooked, 6 oz. (180 g)	0.2

Fish

Salmon, sockeye, cooked, 3 oz. (90 g)	0.2
Tuna, canned and drained, 3 oz. (90 g)	0.4

Cereals

100% bran cereal, 1/2 cup (125 ml)	0.5
Cereal, whole grain flakes, 2/3 cup (160 ml)	0.5

Fruits and vegetables

Avocado, Florida, 1/2 medium	0.4
Avocado, California, 1/2 medium	0.2
Banana, 1 medium	0.7
Potato, baked, 1 medium w/ skin	0.7

What about a vitamin B6 supplement?

If you're feeling blue and you'd like to try a supplement, reach for 50 to 100 milligrams of vitamin B6 once a day. This is the amount that's been used in the research studies done to date. However, you need to know that taking only one B vitamin in high doses can upset your body's balance, because all the B vitamins work together (there are eight different B vitamins). For this reason I recommend using a B-complex supplement that contains all of the Bs—I suggest a supplement that contains 50 to 100 milligrams of B6. If you do decide to take vitamin B6 alone, don't take more than 100 milligrams per day. Too much vitamin B6 taken over a period of time can cause irreversible nerve damage.

herbal remedies

DEPRESSION AND ST. JOHN'S WORT

St. John's Wort (*Hypericum perforatum*) is a yellow-flowered plant that has been heralded for centuries for its ability to balance emotions. In its modern, standardized form, it has been widely used for years in Europe to treat both mild depression and

Seasonal Affective Disorder (SAD), a mood disorder related to the absence of light during the winter. In 1997, British researchers analyzed 26 controlled studies involving in 1,700 patients. The report concluded that the herb was as *effective as certain antidepressant drugs* in treating mild to moderate depression. There's no question in my mind that the evidence for this herb's effectiveness is strong and convincing.

Scientists are still trying to determine exactly how this herbal remedy works. Many experts believe that St. John's Wort acts to keep brain serotonin levels high for longer periods of time than usual, just like the popular antidepressant drugs Paxil®, Zoloft®, and Prozac®.

The power of St. John's Wort lies in two active ingredients, called hypericin and hyperforin. Researchers today attribute much of the herb's effectiveness to hyperforin. A large German study has found that people who take a St. John's Wort extract containing a higher amount of hyperforin report better improvement in symptoms than when they take an extract containing a lesser amount. In fact, 70 percent of study participants reported their depression was much or very much improved after using the high hyperforin content St. John's Wort. High hyperforin content in a St. John's Wort extract has also been shown to cause greater brain wave activity, providing more evidence that it's hyperforin, not hypericin, that influences serotonin levels.[7]

Maybe you're wondering what all this science talk has to do with you. Well, the research results should guide you when it comes to buying a St. John's Wort supplement at your local health food store. As I've said before, I always try to recommend herbal extracts that have been backed by scientific study. In the case of St. John's Wort, you want to look for a product standardized to contain 0.3 percent hypericin, and at least 3 percent hyperforin.

There are some advanced St. John's Wort formulas now on the market, and one in particular, called Movana™, has been used in clinical studies. It contains a guaranteed minimum of 3 percent hyperforin!

To receive full benefits from St. John's Wort, you need to take 300 milligrams of standardized extract three times daily. The herb has a strong record of safety. However, in a few cases it has been reported to cause sensitivity to sunlight in very light-skinned individuals. It can be used during pregnancy and breast-feeding. I don't advise that you start taking St. John's Wort if you're currently on antidepressant therapy. Under your physician's guidance, it is possible to taper off your use of Paxil®, Prozac®, or Zoloft® and at the same time gradually increase the herb dose while decreasing the drug dose.

If you're taking any other antidepressant drug, do not take it concurrently with St. John's Wort. You must wait a week or two after stopping the medication before taking the herb. Always consult your physician first before stopping use of any medication.

ANXIETY AND KAVA KAVA

Perhaps it's not mild depression that's plaguing you. Perhaps rather than feeling blue, you're experiencing increased nervousness, restlessness, and the feeling that something is wrong. Increased anxiety is a mood change often reported by perimenopausal women. Anxiety is described by psychologists as a feeling of apprehension, uncertainty, and fear. It's also associated with physical changes—increased heart rate, sweating, and even tremors. Anxiety can sometimes cause insomnia, or make existing sleep problems worse.

That being said, enter the latest herbal remedy to hit the market: kava kava (*Piper methysticum*). This herbal elixir is extracted from the roots of the South Pacific kava shrub. The use of kava kava predates written history in this area. Europeans first documented the kava drinking ceremonies of Polynesian peoples in the 18th century. Kava drinkers experienced greater tranquility and sociability, and an overall calming, relaxing effect. If the drink was strong enough the user went to sleep. Kava does not, however, produce a hangover. Today, kava extract is used in low doses to soothe the nerves without interfering with alertness, and in higher doses it's an effective sleeping aid.

Experts believe that kava's active ingredients, called kavalactones, exert their effect by acting on the limbic system of the brain, the centre of our emotions. Research has found kava to have therapeutic value in treating anxiety. One double blind study using a standardized kava extract confirmed the herb's effectiveness by measuring its anti-anxiety effect with the Hamilton Anxiety Scale, a standard test used by psychiatrists to measure anxiety levels. Another study found that menopausal women with anxiety disorders obtained significant relief from kava after just one week; relief levels reached their plateau after one month. Women in the study did not experience the negative side effects caused by traditional drugs like Valium®.[8]

According to the research the most effective kava extracts are standardized to contain 30 percent kavalactones. The dosages of kava extracts used in the studies deliver anywhere from 60 to 120 milligrams of kavalactones daily. For most products, this translates into one to three tablets or capsules daily. Start with one standardized tablet.

If you find this doesn't help your symptoms, increase the dose, up to a maximum of three tablets or capsules daily.

Kava has a wide margin of safety. Users to date have experienced very low incidence of side effects, which may include mild stomach upset, headaches, or dizziness. The German Commission E advises consumers not to take kava for longer than three months without medical advice. This recommendation probably reflects the fact that clinical studies on the safety and effectiveness of long-term kava use have not yet been done.

THE bottom LINE...

Leslie's recommendations for preventing mood swings

1   Eat three meals each day plus one or two snacks. My general rule is to go no longer than four to five hours without eating during the day. If there's a longer gap than this between your meals, plan for a between-meal snack.

2   Eat between 5 and 12 servings of grain foods and 5 to 10 fruit and vegetable servings each day to ensure you get enough carbohydrate in your diet.

3   Eliminate caffeine containing beverages and foods. Caffeine increases anxiety and irritability in some individuals.

4   Get more omega-3 fats into your diet. Eat fish three times each week. Make sure at least one-half of your added fats and oils are rich in the omega-3 fat called alpha-linolenic acid, or ALA (i.e. two out of four teaspoons or 10 out of 20 millilitres).

5   Eliminate alcoholic beverages, which can worsen feelings of depression.

6   Make sure you're getting enough vitamin B6 in your diet, since this nutrient is needed to convert the amino acid tryptophan to serotonin.

7   If you suffer from mild depression and you're already eating well and taking a multivitamin and mineral pill, try a daily 50- or 100-milligram B6 supplement. If you're not taking a multivitamin and mineral supplement, take a B complex supplement every day (check the ingredients to make sure it gives you 50 to 100 milligrams of B6).

8   If you've tried B6 and it didn't help your depression, take a standardized extract of St. John's Wort. Take 300 milligrams three times daily. Make sure to buy a product that is standardized to contain 0.3 percent hypericin and 3 percent hyperforin. Movana™ is one such product.

9   If you're experiencing anxiety or panic attacks, try kava kava. Buy a product standardized to contain 30 percent kavalactones. Take one to three capsules a day, or enough that you get 60 to 120 milligrams of kavalactones daily. Don't use kava kava for more than three months at a time without consulting your physician.

10 If your mood swings do not improve with dietary changes or the recommended supplements, consult your doctor. Serious emotional problems may require medication. If perimenopausal mood changes take over your life, a psychologist can also be helpful in helping you discover the underlying causes of your stress and teaching you new techniques for coping with it.

forgetfulness and fuzzy thinking

"I have always thought my mind was pretty sharp. For the last year or so, my brain has become like peach fuzz. I have difficulty remembering the names of people I worked with less than a year ago; I constantly misplace things; I go into a room and can't remember why I was going there. It's very frustrating."

4

Can't remember where you left your wallet? Or perhaps your next door neighbour's name has recently eluded you at the most embarrassing possible moment? We've all had memory lapses at one time or another. But there is also a definite link between brain power and hormonal fluctuations. If you have children, think back to the last time you were pregnant. If you're like many of my friends, you probably felt that your brain had turned to mush. Well, going through perimenopause can affect your ability to think and concentrate in the same way. Fortunately, this mid-life brain drain is temporary. You won't continue to forget simple things (like your phone number) forever.

Sometimes other things besides perimenopausal hormonal fluctations may contribute to forgetfulness. For starters, we have to face the fact that there's an aging process at work. The older we get, the more short-term memory we lose. That goes for both women and men. Finnish researchers studied 70 women between the ages of 47 and 65, and found that the results of most tests of mental performance were correlated with age. Older women were slower, and made more mistakes than younger women. When these women were given estrogen replacement therapy for three months (short-term use), their cognitive abilities did not improve.[1] It seems that a little memory loss is a natural part of aging.

Menopausal symptoms can cause memory problems too. Certainly insomnia and fatigue can reduce your ability to think clearly. And sometimes the stress of experiencing physical changes or emotional turmoil related to menopause can affect your mental performance.

When it comes to hormonal changes, scientists have collected a fair amount of evidence that shows that estrogen affects aspects of brain chemistry and structure that are important for memory, and that the loss of estrogen associated with menopause may be largely responsible for the decline in memory that some women experience in their later years. Scientists have theorized that estrogen is needed for the transfer of nerve messages to specific regions in the brain.

Does all this mean that estrogen replacement therapy might help preserve memory and prevent senility? Some controlled studies demonstrate that estrogen use in menopausal women enhances short- and long-term memory and increases the capacity to learn new material. An overview of ten observational studies of post-menopausal estrogen use published in the *Journal of the American Medical Association* (these were not placebo-controlled trials) suggests that women on estrogen therapy have a 29 percent lower risk of developing dementia than those who don't use supplemental estrogen. Studies have also found estrogen use to be associated with a lower risk of Alzheimer's disease. Since June 1997, four controlled trials have investigated the effect of estrogen in women with Alzheimer's disease. Although the results look promising, many of these studies were either small, of short duration, or poorly controlled.[2]

At this stage in the game, it's too soon to say that estrogen therapy prevents a decline in mental prowess, or prevents dementia. Until well controlled, larger, longer studies give us clearer answers, there are a few things you can do right now to sharpen your thinking and slow down the aging of your brain.

dietary approaches

EAT BREAKFAST EVERY DAY

Parents tell their children to eat breakfast time and time again. Well, what's good for kids is good for you, too. Many studies of both children and adults have shown that compared to breakfast eaters, individuals who skip the morning meal do not score as well on tests of mental performance that same morning. Breakfast skipping appears to affect recall and memory tasks more than any other cognitive function.[3] One reason we don't perform well without breakfast is that after a night of sleeping we wake up in a fasting state. That means our blood glucose (blood sugar) levels are low—and blood glucose supplies energy to the brain. Breakfast foods supply carbohydrates that are converted to glucose in the bloodstream, and supply the energy needed for peak mental performance.

Breakfast also supplies key nutrients, including important B vitamins, iron, and calcium. Research has shown that when we skip breakfast, we usually don't manage to catch up later in the day on our intake of the nutrients we missed.

So what's the best breakfast? I recommend having some carbohydrate to elevate blood glucose and a little protein to help sustain energy levels longer. Eating protein has this effect partly because it takes longer to digest. As a result, the carbohydrate you eat with protein is converted to glucose more slowly. In a sense, by eating a little protein with the carbohydrate, you are giving yourself "time release" energy, rather than sharply elevating your blood glucose all at once. Following are a few breakfast ideas that meet my criteria—and also help you meet your daily calcium and vitamin C requirements:

- Whole grain cereal with low fat milk or calcium-fortified soy beverage. Top with fruit or have a small glass of citrus juice. To increase your fibre intake, choose a breakfast cereal that contains at least 4 grams of fibre per serving. The nutrition information panel will give you the cereal's fibre content.
- Whole grain toast with a poached or hard-boiled egg and a fruit salad.
- Homemade breakfast smoothie made with a calcium-fortified soy beverage, orange juice, and a banana. Add soy protein isolate powder or egg whites for a protein boost.
- In a hurry? If you usually eat breakfast running out the door, grab a piece of fruit, a cereal bar, and a low fat yogurt for protein (and calcium). You might not be able to eat the yogurt in the car or on the bus, but you can certainly eat it when you get to work.

HIGH PROTEIN AT MIDDAY

Many of my clients complain that they feel sleepy or lethargic after lunch. If you want to be sharp and feel more energetic, try eating protein, vegetables, and fruit. Here's why.

The body breaks down protein-rich foods like meat, poultry, and fish into smaller units called amino acids. Amino acids are the body's building blocks for making muscle, hormones, enzymes, and brain chemicals called neurotransmitters. If you've read Chapter 3, on mood swings, then you already know all about neurotransmitters. If not, check the chapter out. A high protein meal causes a rise in blood levels of a specific amino acid called tyrosine. Once in the brain, tyrosine is converted to the neurotransmitters called dopamine and norepinephrine. These neurotransmitters have been found to improve alertness, sharpen thinking, and enhance energy levels.

What does a high protein lunch look like? Here are a few examples of what might fit the bill:

- Large green salad with 3 to 4 ounces (90 to 120 grams) of tuna or grilled chicken, glass of milk or soy beverage, piece of fruit.
- Stir-fried chicken or tofu with plenty of vegetables, a piece of fruit, water.
- Omelet served with a green salad or steamed vegetables, fruit salad, water.

I'll often grill an extra piece of fish or chicken at dinner and bring it to work with me for lunch the next day. I'll also steam extra vegetables at dinner and enjoy them the next day cold, or I'll serve the protein on a bed of greens. Keep in mind through, that a high protein lunch doesn't give you enough energy to carry you through the rest of the day. You will need a snack to boost your blood sugar levels about three to four hours after lunch. Even when you eat a starchy lunch, your blood sugar levels normally decline three to four hours later. To prevent that mid-afternoon drop in blood glucose and mental performance, fuel your brain with a snack combining carbohydrate and protein: fruit and yogurt, or whole grain crackers and low fat cheese.

GET MORE OMEGA-3 FATS

As you might have read in Chapter 3, the type of fat we eat is very important for the healthy functioning of our brain. A large proportion of the communicating membranes of the brain is made up of two omega-3 fats, docosahexaenoic acid (DHA) and eicosapentaenoic acid (EPA). Your brain cells must constantly refresh themselves with a new supply of omega-3 fats. When we eat oily fish like salmon, trout, and sardines, we get a good supply of EPA and DHA. But these two omega-3 fats can also be made inside the body from another omega-3 fat called alpha-linolenic acid (ALA). ALA is plentiful in flaxseed oil, canola oil, and walnut oil. It's called an essential fatty acid because it's essential to our health *and* our bodies cannot make it—it must be supplied by our diet.

While most Canadians likely eat too much fat, experts are concerned that we may not be getting enough omega-3 fats for optimal brain health. To get more of them into your diet, aim to consume the following:

- Three to six ounces (90 to 180 grams) of fish high in omega-3 oils at least three times a week.
- Use vegetable oils rich in omega-3 fats. Try to get 2 to 3 teaspoons (10 to 15 millilitres) per day of canola, flaxseed, or walnut oil. Corn, sunflower, safflower, and olive oils contain almost no omega-3 fats.

vitamins and minerals

CHOLINE

Although not an official vitamin, choline is a member of the B vitamin family. It's found in egg yolks, organ meats, and legumes. It's one of the building blocks used to manufacture a memory neurotransmitter called acetylcholine. Levels of acetylcholine increase in proportion to the amount of choline in the diet. Choline supplements have been shown to enhance memory and reaction time in animals, particularly aging animals. Researchers currently believe that choline supplements will improve the brain's ability to do its tasks only in people who are actually deficient in the nutrient. Stress and aging can deplete choline levels.

While we don't yet know if supplemental choline will improve memory in people who have normal choline levels, it's still important to get enough of this nutrient in your diet. In fact, in 1998 the Food and Nutrition Board of the National Academy of Sciences, a body consisting of Canadian and American experts, released for the very first time a recommended daily intake for choline. There is evidence that choline may be needed in the diet because the amount synthesized by our body may be insufficient to meet our needs. Healthy women need 425 milligrams of choline each day. The best food sources are egg yolks, liver and other organ meats, brewer's yeast, wheat germ, soybeans, peanuts, and green peas.

If you don't regularly eat egg yolks, organ meats, or legumes, you can get choline from lecithin supplements. The maximum safe dosage is 2,500 milligrams (2.5 grams) of choline per day. Be warned that taking large amounts of choline can cause low blood pressure and a fishy body odour in some people (pass the soybeans please!).

IRON

You're probably familiar with iron's role in preventing anemia. When your diet lacks iron, your red blood cells become less efficient at transporting oxygen to your cells for energy. Eventually your body iron stores run low, and you end up feeling tired and lethargic. At this point a blood test will diagnose iron deficiency anemia. But you might not have realized that iron is also used to make certain brain neurotransmitters, in particular the neurotransmitters that regulate the ability to pay attention. It's important to keep in mind that long before red blood cells are depleted of iron and anemia is diagnosed by a standard blood test, a developing iron deficiency can affect your mental performance. And because of the neurotransmitter link, a deficiency of iron can also directly affect your mood, attention span, and learning ability.

NUTRITION TIP

Pumping iron

To help you stay alert, energetic, and focussed, make a point of adding a few of the following foods to your daily diet—they all top the list when it comes to iron content.

IRON CONTENT OF IRON-RICH FOODS (MILLIGRAMS)

3 oz. (90 g) lean beef	3
I cup (250 ml) beans in tomato sauce	5
1/2 cup (125 ml) kidney beans	2.5
1/2 cup (125 ml) prune juice	5
I cup (250 ml)cooked spinach	4
6 dried apricots	2.8
1/2 cup (125 ml) Cream of Wheat	8
I tbsp. (15 ml) blackstrap molasses	3.2
I tbsp. (15 ml) wheat germ	2.5

If you are still menstruating, you need 13 milligrams of iron each day. After menopause, your need decreases to nine milligrams per day. To help you get more iron into your diet, use my chart, above. Iron in food is classified either as "heme" or "non-heme" iron. Heme iron is very well absorbed by the body—it's the form of iron found in red meat, poultry, and fish. Foods containing significant amounts of non-heme iron include whole grain breads and cereals, fortified breakfast cereals, beans, vegetables, and fruit. This form of iron accounts for 85 percent of our dietary intake of the mineral, but it is less well absorbed. In fact, you'd have to eat four cups of raw spinach to get as much useable iron as you receive from a three-ounce (90 g) serving of lean beef.

Maximizing iron absorption

Fortunately, you can take action to enhance your body's ability to absorb non-heme iron. Practice these tips to get the most from your foods: add some vitamin C with foods rich in non-heme iron (top your whole grain cereal with strawberries or have it with a glass of citrus juice); include a source of heme iron with foods containing non-heme iron (a little meat or chicken tossed into your rice stir-fry will do it); pull out your cast iron cookware; don't drink coffee or tea with an iron-rich meal as the beverages' tannins will prevent iron absorption.

What about a multivitamin supplement?

You're at risk for iron deficiency if any of the following applies to you: you're still menstruating; you engage in heavy endurance exercise; you don't eat animal foods and are unsure about vegetarian iron sources; you're adhering to a low calorie diet.

Look for a "high potency" multivitamin or a "woman's" formula supplement; they should contain between 15 and 18 milligrams of iron. Iron-only supplements should be taken under supervision and only if you have an iron deficiency diagnosed by your physician.

BORON

Scientific evidence suggests that this trace mineral plays an important role in brain function. Studies have shown that boron deficiency results in poor performance in tasks involving neuromuscular speed and dexterity, attention, and short-term memory. Study participants with low boron intakes suffered from significantly poorer performances in test of hand-eye coordination, attention, perception, and memory as opposed to their counterparts with high dietary boron levels. The individuals with lower boron also had significantly less brain electrical activity.

Because boron has not yet been recognized as an essential nutrient for humans, no recommended daily intake has been established. A daily intake of between 1.5 and 3 milligrams is probably more than adequate to meet daily requirements, but we don't really know for sure if this amount is optimal for brain function. The main food sources for boron are fruits and vegetables, but actual content depends on the food's soil. If you want to take a supplement, 3 to 9 milligrams per day is a very safe amount.

herbal remedies

GINGKO

Also known as maidenhair, ginkgo (*Ginkgo biloba*) is one of the most popular herbs to hit the North American market in recent years. Gingko is touted to improve memory loss and slow the progression of Alzheimer's disease. It turns out that the claims are very likely true. Gingko is one of the most heavily researched herbs in the world. The most recent study to make news was a 52-week American trial, in which 309 patients with mild to moderate dementia as a result of Alzheimer's Disease or stroke participated. Patients were given either 40 milligrams of a special standardized gingko extract (called EGb 761) at breakfast, lunch, and dinner, or a placebo pill. After one year the placebo group showed a decline in cognitive function, whereas the group that had received gingko did not show an overall decline. When the researchers looked at the Alzheimer's patients only, they found modest, but significant, improvements in memory and other brain functions.

Gingko extracts are made from the fan shaped, bilobed leaves of the gingko tree, a tree that reaches heights of over 100 feet tall and grows here in North America. Gingko may act in one of two ways to enhance memory. A number of studies suggest that gingko increases circulation and oxygen delivery to the brain. The herb's active ingredients also make blood cells called platelets less sticky. As a result, circulation becomes more efficient.[4] (Gingko also enhances blood flow to the extremities and studies have found the herb to improve sex drive—Chapter 5 has more on this!)

What's more, gingko has a strong antioxidant effect in the brain, the eye, and the cardiovascular system, meaning that it protects these tissues from free radical damage. Free radical damage to brain cells is widely accepted as a contributing factor in Alzheimer's disease. Free radicals are unstable oxygen molecules that seek electrons from other molecules and in the process, cause cellular damage. Free radicals can damage brain cells, the genetic material of cells, protein molecules in the eye, and cell membranes. Any compound that is able to neutralize these harmful free radicals is called an antioxidant. (For more on free radicals and antioxidants, see page 145 in Chapter 9.) Antioxidant compounds, be it vitamin C in oranges, lycopene in tomatoes, or active compounds in gingko biloba, essentially "mop up" free radicals and as a result, protect our cells from damage. Scientists aren't sure if gingko's positive effect on brain function is largely due to its antioxidant ability to prevent damage to brain cells, or its power to increase blood flow to the brain.

Although no studies have been done in perimenopausal or post-menopausal women, I do recommend gingko to my clients to help reduce the effects of aging on brain cells. Researchers have identified the active compounds that appear responsible for gingko's beneficial effects. They are called terpene lactones and gingko flavone glycosides. Guidelines for buying a top quality gingko supplement are as follows:

- Choose a product that is standardized to contain 24 percent gingko flavone glycosides and 6 percent terpene lactones.
- The EGb 761 extract used in the scientific research is sold as Ginkoba® in Canada and the United States.

The research indicates that the effective daily dose is between 120 and 240 milligrams, taken in two to three doses over the day. Start with the lower 120-milligram dose by taking a 40-milligram tablet with three meals. Ginkgo is safe to use during pregnancy and breast-feeding, and there are no known interactions with other medications. On rare occasions gingko may cause gastrointestinal upset, headache, or an allergic skin reaction in susceptible individuals. In that case, lower your dosage, and if symptoms persist, discontinue use. You may then want to consult with your physician or other qualified health care practitioner to determine if any other herbal remedies may be of use to you.

THE bottom LINE...

Leslie's recommendations for improving memory

1   Eat breakfast every day to provide your brain cells with their preferred fuel source—carbohydrate. To sustain your blood glucose levels, make sure your breakfast includes both carbohydrate and protein.

2   To stay alert and focussed in the afternoon, try a high protein lunch. A meal consisting of chicken or fish and plenty of vegetables provides your brain with more tyrosine, an amino acid used to produce brain chemicals that increase alertness.

3   Make sure the fats and oils you add to your diet come mainly from the omega-3 family. These special fats are used by the body to manufacture a large part of the communicating membranes of the brain. Eat fish at least three times per week. Use flaxseed oil, canola oil, and walnut oil more often. Eat more soyfoods, omega-3 eggs, and green leafy vegetables.

4   To help your brain manufacture more of the memory neurotransmitter acetyl-choline, increase your intake of foods rich in choline, a fat-like member of the B vitamin family. Good sources are eggs, legumes, and organ meats. If these foods aren't on your A-list, consider taking a choline or lecithin supplement.

5   Reach for iron-rich foods every day. Remember, your body uses iron to make brain chemicals that regulate your ability to pay attention. It you're at risk for iron deficiency, be sure to take a multivitamin and mineral supplement that includes between 15 and 18 milligrams of the mineral.

6   Be sure to eat 5 to 10 servings of fruits and vegetables each day to help you get more boron for brain function. While there is no official recommended intake for this trace mineral, it's extremely safe to use a supplement; try adding 3 to 9 milligrams to your daily diet.

7   Even though it might not improve a healthy woman's short term memory, a standardized extract of gingko biloba probably will protect your brain cells from the ravages of aging. Look for an extract that contains 24 percent gingko flavone glycosides. Take one 40-milligram tablet with breakfast, lunch, and dinner.

sexual changes

"I can't say that my interest in sex changed when going through menopause. I can say, though, that my dryness made it uncomfortable to the point of not enjoying it."

5

For women who are accustomed to enjoying regular sexual activity, experiencing sexual symptoms due to menopause can be one of the most disconcerting aspects of this life cycle transition. Current estimates indicate that somewhere between 20 and 45 percent of peri- and post-menopausal women report vaginal dryness—they take longer to become lubricated during sexual arousal and intercourse may become uncomfortable. During the perimenopausal years, vaginal dryness is often a transient condition that improves as estrogen levels increase again.

Vaginal dryness is caused by a decline in estrogen levels. As estrogen levels fall, the walls of the vagina become smaller, thinner, and less elastic. Secretion of the fluids that naturally protect the vagina from infection and lubricate it for sexual intercourse also decreases. Lack of lubrication, in turn, can make intercourse painful and cause bleeding and soreness. Regular sexual intercourse can actually help prevent these problems by stretching the vagina and increasing its blood supply and lubrication.

Popular beliefs hold that with menopause comes a loss of interest in sex. While researchers have not found a link between estrogen levels and libido, many women do complain that their sex drive lessens around the time of menopause. Sometimes decreased sexual desire is the result of menopausal symptoms that interfere with sexual intercourse. Libido, or sex drive, is really a function of your brain. Certainly vaginal dryness, hot flashes, night sweats, and insomnia can contribute to a temporary lack of interest in sex.

Androgen (male) hormones, such as testosterone, may also be a factor. These hormones activate specific receptors in the brain to turn on sexual desire. Women who have had hysterectomies report being less interested in sex more often than women who experience natural menopause. Studies in women who have experienced premature menopause have led researchers to theorize that a lack of testosterone due to decreased production in the ovaries may cause some menopausal libido problems. In fact, a number of studies have found that adding testosterone to estrogen replacement therapy improves sexual motivation and desire.[1] While estrogen therapy alone is effective at relieving vaginal dryness, it is less effective at enhancing sexual desire and arousal. Other medical doctors attribute a decline in progesterone production to be largely responsible for decreased libido experienced around menopause. While little research has been done in this area, the use of progesterone creams and oils is becoming more popular (see the discussion on page 58).

So what does all this mean? Well you certainly don't have to give up sex just because you've entered your "change of life." A healthy sexual relationship with someone you care for deeply is very important for emotional well being. If you are experiencing serious libido problems, talk to your doctor about the possibility of hormonal therapy. If you're troubled by vaginal dryness there are several things you can do on your own to minimize and possibly alleviate this condition.

dietary approaches

SOY FOODS AND ISOFLAVONES

If you read Chapter 1, on hot flashes, then you're already an expert on soy foods. Studies show that soy's natural plant estrogens, called isoflavones, can improve vaginal dryness as well as reduce hot flashes. Finnish and Israeli researchers have looked at the effect a phytoestrogen-rich diet has on hot flashes and vaginal dryness. In a study involving 145 women with menopausal symptoms, participants were randomly assigned to eat either a diet that contained 25 percent of its calories from phytoestrogen-rich foods (including tofu, soy beverages, miso, and flaxseed) or their regular diet. After 12 weeks, blood levels of phytoestrogens had increased significantly in women eating the diet rich in soy foods, but remained unchanged in the women eating their regular diet. Reductions in hot flashes and vaginal dryness scores were more significant in the women assigned the phytoestrogen-rich diet. Other studies have also shown that post-menopausal women report improved vaginal lubrication when regularly eating soy foods.[2]

How can soy reverse vaginal dryness? The natural isoflavone compounds in soybeans are able to bind to estrogen receptors in the vagina and exert a weak estrogen-like effect. Acting like estrogen, although much less potent, soy's isoflavones can increase the thickness and elasticity of the vaginal walls, as well as increase vaginal secretions.

Going nuts with soy

You may already have noticed that soy "nuts" (roasted soybeans) provide you with one of the easiest ways to get your phytoestrogens. With soy nuts, you certainly get the most isoflavones for the smallest amount of food. And if you're worried about extra fat and calories, rest assured, there's no need to fret. Soy nuts have less than half the fat found in actual nuts. One ounce (1/4 cup or 50 millilitres) of plain roasted soy nuts delivers 136 calories, 6 grams of fat (only 1 gram is saturated), 10 grams of soy protein, and 5 grams of fibre. Compare that to the same amount of peanuts, which packs 170 calories, 14 grams of fat, 7 grams of protein, and 3 grams of fibre. On all nutrition scores, soy nuts come out the winner.

- Snack on soy nuts right from the bag.
- Sprinkle them over your green salads.
- Sprinkle them over a bowl of frozen yogurt.
- Stir soy nuts into stir fried dishes along with vegetables and tofu, chicken, or lean meat.
- Add them to a bowl of your favourite hot breakfast cereal.
- Create a homemade snack mix with soy nuts, shredded wheat squares, raisins, dried cranberries, and low fat granola.

How much soy do you need?

In Chapter 1, on hot flashes, I recommended an intake of 50 to 90 milligrams of isoflavones each day. Many experts believe that this is the amount of phytoestrogens needed to achieve the desired effects.

In Chapter 1 you'll find 10 suggestions for adding isoflavones to your diet, 10 ways to increase your soy intake, and a dictionary of soy foods, that demystifies what soy products are and how to use them (see pages 6–12). In Appendix 3, you'll also find some tasty recipes that will help you experiment with soy in the kitchen. To ensure a daily dose of at least 50 milligrams of isoflavones, I recommend you also try one of the following strategies:

- Every morning, enjoy a breakfast smoothie made with a soy beverage, fruit, and soy protein isolate powder (see page 11 for a list of high quality brands).
- Add 2 tablespoons (30 millilitres) of soy protein isolate powder to your morning orange juice (not nearly as tasty, although I have a few clients who do this religiously).
- Munch on 1/4 cup (50 millilitres) of roasted soy "nuts" as a regular midday snack. You'll find these nuts at health food stores. They come in plain or flavoured varieties. They're quite tasty and don't worry, they contain less fat than actual nuts. Just stick to a small serving!

Do isoflavone pills work?

Unfortunately, I'm afraid not. At this time, the research shows that they're not effective in reducing menopausal symptoms. It seems there's something special about getting your isoflavones along with the protein and other natural components of soy foods. You'd better pull out that blender!

WATER AND FLUIDS

I can't emphasize enough the importance of drinking enough fluids. Keeping your whole body adequately hydrated at all times is a critical component of a healthy lifestyle. We all know the effects of dehydration—dry skin, chapped lips, and lower energy levels. Well, a lack of fluids can affect your vagina in the same way. Dehydration decreases natural body secretions and can exacerbate vaginal dryness caused by an estrogen deficiency. You must drink enough water every day! There's no magic behind that "eight glasses of water per day" recommendation. To maintain fluid balance, you need to drink at least two to three litres of fluid daily, and that translates into 8 to 12 8 ounce (250 millilitres) glasses. If you exercise, if you work in an air-conditioned building, or if you spend time outside in hot, humid weather, then you need *more* than 8 to 12 glasses. Water, vegetable juice, unsweetened fruit juice, milk, herbal tea, soup, and high water content fruits and vegetables all contribute to your daily fluid intake—but to be sure you're getting enough, always drink at least eight glasses of water daily. Avoid caffeine and alcohol, which can cause your body to lose water.

herbal remedies

ASIAN (PANAX) GINSENG

If you've ever been to a health food store in search of an energy boost, chances are you've come across ginseng. Among the top five selling herbal remedies in North America, *Panax ginseng* (Asian, Korean, and Chinese) is best known for its ability to help the body deal with stress. Probably because it helps them deal better with stress, users report that they experience more consistent energy levels. Now it also appears that the health benefits of ginseng may include improving vaginal dryness associated with menopause. One study reported in the *British Journal of Medicine* found that *Panax* ginseng had a protective effect on vaginal tissue in post-menopausal women. Women who took the herb for six weeks noticed an improvement in vaginal dryness.[3] Ginseng does not have an estrogenic effect. Rather, it encourages the pituitary gland to increase the body's production of hormones that affect vaginal tissue.

RESEARCH FILE

Gingko for better sex?

What will those scientists decide to study next? After a patient taking gingko biloba for memory problems reported improved erections, California researchers decided to investigate whether there was any substance to the patient's story. Each day, they gave from 60 to 120 milligrams of standardized gingko extract to a group of 63 men and women who complained of sexual dysfunction as a result of using antidepressant medication. And guess what? Gingko was found to be 84 percent effective in treating sexual dysfunction. Women were more responsive than men, with a success rate of 91 percent versus the men's rate of 76 percent.[4] It appears that gingko's ability to increase blood and oxygen delivery to the tissues may not only help your brain function better, but might also improve your sex life as well!

Ginseng's benefits can be attributed to active compounds called ginsenosides. Two in particular, Rg1 and Rb1, have received the most attention from researchers and most studies have focused on ginseng extracts standardized to contain four to seven percent ginsenosides. When buying ginseng, look for a statement of standardization, or better yet, choose a product stating "G115" on the label. This designation indicates that the product contains a special extract of ginsenosides that has been used in research. The usual daily dosage of a standardized extract is 100 or 200 milligrams once daily. Take ginseng in cycles—two to three weeks on, one week off. Some experts believe that over time, your body can get used to the effects of ginseng, and its effectiveness is then reduced. Taking it in cycles helps prevent this problem. According to the German Commission E, ginseng is safe to use for up to three months at a time in the cyclical way described.

Ginseng is relatively safe at the 100 or 200 milligram dosage. In some people, it may cause mild stomach upset, irritability, and insomnia. To avoid overstimulation, start with 100 milligrams a day. If you experience overstimulation at this dose, avoid using caffeine while you're on ginseng. Ginseng should not be used during pregnancy or breast-feeding, and it's not suitable for individuals with uncontrolled high blood pressure. There have also been a few reports of ginseng causing spotting in post-menopausal women. If you experience this side effect, stop taking the herb. If spotting continues, consult your physician.

SIBERIAN GINSENG

Siberian ginseng (*Eleutherococcus senticosus*) has much milder effects than *Panax*, or Asian, ginseng, and few reported side effects. Pregnant and nursing women can safely take Siberian ginseng and it's much less likely to cause overstimulation in sensitive individuals. But keep in mind that in the research we have to date, the type of ginseng shown to improve vaginal cell maturation is *Panax* ginseng, not Siberian.

To ensure that you are buying a high quality extract, choose one standardized to contain eleutherosides B and E. The usual dosage is 300 to 400 milligrams once daily for six to eight weeks, followed by a one to two week break. It is safe to use Siberian ginseng for up to three months, and also safe to take repeated courses of the herb.

DONG QUAI

Dong quai (*Angelica sinensis*) is often recommended by herbalists as an all-purpose herb for gynecological complaints, including menopausal symptoms. However, if you're taking this herb to treat hot flashes or vaginal dryness, you might want to give it a second thought. When researchers from the Kaiser Permanente Medical Center in Oakland, California assessed the herb's effects in 71 post-menopausal women over 24 weeks, they found no difference between the groups taking dong quai or placebo with respect to vaginal wall thickness, rate of vaginal cell maturation, or hot flashes. The researchers concluded that when used alone, dong quai does not have an estrogen-like effect on vaginal tissues and is no more helpful than placebo in relieving menopausal symptoms.[5]

The results of this study are a little surprising, given dong quai's long tradition of use in Asia. However, practitioners of Traditional Chinese Medicine (TCM) usually prescribe dong quai in combination with other herbs. While the herb might not reduce certain menopausal symptoms all by itself, it might work as part of a combination of herbs. If you're interested in learning more about dong quai, I recommend you consult a practitioner well trained in the use of traditional Chinese herbs.

other ways to prevent vaginal dryness

In addition to the dietary and herbal suggestions I've provided, here are some other ways to combat vaginal dryness:

1   Use a vaginal lubricant. Many women find that vaginal lubricants (gels and liquids) replenish moisture to the vaginal lining and eliminate general itchiness and discomfort during sexual intercourse. If you decide to try an external lubricant, be sure to buy a water-based product such as Replens®, Vagisil®, Gyne-Moistrin™, or KY Long Lasting Vaginal Moisturizer®. Water-based lubricants are less likely to cause bacterial growth or infection than oil-based products.

    Depending on the severity of vaginal dryness, these products may be used anywhere from daily to once every three days.

2   Try vitamin E suppositories. These suppositories can be made by a compounding pharmacist (to find such a pharmacist in your community, contact the College of Pharmacists in your province). Each suppository will contain 120 international units (IU) of vitamin E. After insertion into the vagina, the suppository softens and dissolves in the cavity. Some vitamin E will be absorbed into the body through the vaginal lining, but most of the oil based vitamin will act to lubricate the vagina. Vitamin E suppositories can be used once daily or as needed.

NATURAL PROGESTERONE REPLACEMENT?

Natural progesterone creams contain progesterone synthesized in the laboratory from active compounds found in wild yams called diosgenins and is identical in structure to that made by your body. Proponents of natural progesterone state that is safer than the progestins prescribed in hormone replacement therapy.

Little has been done to assess the effectiveness of this type of product, but some of my clients have reported improvement of hot flashes and vaginal dryness with their use.

Some things to keep in mind: natural progesterone creams are available by prescription and should only be used under medical supervision; proper manufacturing is important, so only buy creams from a knowledgeable pharmacist who has experience compounding them; apply cream to areas of thin skin—palms, face, neck, upper chest, inner arms, and thighs—and remember to change the application site regularly; use 1/8 to 1/2 of a teaspoon of cream per application as directed; check with your doctor, pharmacist, or naturopathic physician for detailed dosages information pertaining to your individual situation.

THE bottom LINE...

Leslie's recommendations for minimizing vaginal dryness

1   Start adding soy foods to your daily diet. Once you find a few of these foods that you like, aim to consume at least 50 milligrams of isoflavones from a combination of these foods each day.

2   If soy foods aren't for you, try a protein powder made from isolated soy protein, preferably made from Supro® soy protein isolate. Add soy protein powder to a breakfast milkshake or glass of juice.

3   Be sure to consume enough fluids. Aim to drink at least 8 to 12 glasses of water each day. Avoid beverages and medications that cause your body to lose water. Dehydration can make vaginal dryness worse.

4   Consider trying a daily dose of 100 to 200 milligrams of *Panax* ginseng to help restore vaginal epithelial tissue. Buy a standardized extract containing 4 to 7 percent ginsenosides or look for the G115 statement on the label. Remember to take ginseng in cyclical fashion, two to three weeks on, one week off.

5   Vitamin E suppositories and other vaginal lubricants are also helpful in providing moisture.

menstrual cycle changes

"My periods became a real worry. I'd never had such heavy flow before. On a few occasions, I felt so drained I could barely make it through the day. Thankfully, this didn't go on too long."

6

More than 75 percent of women will experience some change to their monthly cycle during their mid to late 40s or early 50s and this is often the first sign that menopause is approaching. A number of years before her "last" period, a woman may notice that her cycle becomes less frequent or that periods arrive closer together. And often her period shortens in duration as estrogen production fluctuates. While an erratic menstrual cycle can be annoying, what's more distressing is the heavy bleeding that can occur during the perimenopausal years.

Heavy bleeding in perimenopausal women is usually the result of an imbalance of estrogen and progesterone. When ovulation does not occur and your ovaries don't release an egg, progesterone is not produced. Since progesterone normally counters the effects of estrogen, this means that in its absence, estrogen is allowed to continue to build up the uterine lining throughout the month beyond normal limits. The lining becomes very thick and therefore laden with more capillaries than usual, and releases a great deal of blood when it is finally shed at your next period (a naturally orchestrated, sharp decline in both estrogen and progesterone each month catalyzes menstrual bleeding). As your estrogen levels decline with approaching menopause, heavy bleeding will become less of an issue.

While heavy bleeding is a common symptom during the years leading up to menopause, it can still be scary. In some cases, heavy bleeding can also be a sign of something else going on in the uterus—polyps, a fibroid, or less commonly, cancer. Always alert your gynecologist if your periods last more than seven days, if you bleed between your periods, or if your menstrual flow becomes much heavier than usual.

Heavy menstrual bleeding may cause you to experience chills, dizziness, fatigue, and anemia caused by blood loss. To minimize these side effects, make sure you pay attention to your diet.

dietary approaches

GET ENOUGH IRON

Now, more than ever, it's important to eat a diet rich in iron. Iron is used by red blood cells to form hemoglobin, the molecule that transports oxygen from your lungs to all your cells. If your diet is deficient in iron, or if your body loses iron faster than your diet can replace it, red blood cell levels drop and less oxygen is delivered to your tissues. Symptoms of iron deficiency include weakness, lethargy, and fatigue on exertion. Iron deficiency is a progressive condition, which means that even if your iron stores aren't low enough to warrant a formal diagnosis of anemia, you can still be deficient and feel symptoms.

While you're still menstruating, you need 13 milligrams of iron each day. In Chapter 4 I mentioned iron's role in your ability to think and pay attention, and discussed ways to increase your intake. You may remember that iron in food comes in two forms—heme iron and non-heme iron. Heme iron is the form most efficiently absorbed and is found in red meat, chicken, eggs, and fish. Non-heme iron comes from plant foods like whole grains, legumes (lentils, chickpeas, kidney beans), fruit, and vegetables. The body has a harder time absorbing non-heme iron from foods. Eating foods rich in vitamin C along with food sources of non-heme iron will allow your body to absorb much more of the non-heme iron. If you include a little heme iron (for example, meat) with your meal, you'll also increase the absorption of non-heme iron. As you can see by the numbers on page 46, the best iron sources are lean beef, tofu, legumes, enriched breakfast cereals, whole grain breads, raisins, dried apricots, prune juice, spinach, and peas.

What about iron supplements?

To ensure you get 13 milligrams of iron each day, a multivitamin and mineral supplement is a wise idea. Most formulas provide 10 milligrams, but you can find multivitamins that provide up to 18. If you're experiencing persistent heavy bleeding, however, the recommended daily intake of 13 milligrams might not be enough to meet your needs. Sometimes 100 milligrams of supplemental iron daily is needed to rebuild your iron stores. Because iron is toxic in large doses, you should take iron pills only if your doctor has determined that you have low enough iron levels to warrant this level of supplementation. If you are advised to use an iron supplement, take it on an empty stomach to enhance absorption. Many people find that taking their iron supplement just before going to bed reduces stomach upset. Iron can be constipating, so I recommend that you boost your fibre and your water intake when using an iron supplement.

NUTRITION TIP

Boosting your fibre intake

Here are 10 strategies for boosting your fibre intake that are easy to implement, and increase your intake of tasty and healthy foods to boot.

1　Strive to consume five or more servings of fruits and vegetables each day.

2　Eat the skin of the fruits and vegetables you consume whenever possible.

3　Eat at least five servings of whole grain foods each day.

4　Buy higher fibre breakfast cereals. Aim for at least 4 grams of fibre per serving. (Check the nutrition information panel to find out how much fibre the cereal contains.)

5　If you're looking for a real fibre boost at breakfast, choose a 100 percent bran cereal that packs in 10 grams of fibre per half-cup (125 millilitre) serving.

6　Top your breakfast cereal with dried apricots, berries, or raisins.

7　Add two tablespoons (25 millilitres) of natural wheat bran or oat bran to hot cereals, yogurt, casseroles, and soup.

8　Eat legumes more often—add white kidney beans to pasta sauce, black beans to tacos, chickpeas to salads, lentils to soup.

9　Add a handful of nuts, seeds, and raisins to salads.

10　Reach for high fibre snacks like popcorn, dried apricots, or dried or fresh dates.

herbal remedies

CHASTE TREE BERRIES

Extracts of the berries of the Mediterranean chaste tree (*Vitex agnus-castus*) plant have been used in Europe for over 40 years for female menstrual cycle disorders and menopausal complaints. The herb was first mentioned as a medicinal plant some 2,000 years ago when a Greek physician noted the ability of a drink made from the plants' seeds to reduce sexual desire. The herb was also reported to help medieval monks keep their vow of chastity. Accordingly, its Latin name, *agnus castus*, means chaste lamb. Today, the herb is most often used in women with PMS, but chaste berry may also help women manage heavy or frequently occurring periods.

Chaste tree berry contains about 0.5 percent volatile oils along with two compounds called agnuside and aucubin. Studies have shown that an extract of chaste tree berries is able to lower blood levels of a hormone called prolactin. Scientists aren't certain how chaste tree berries do this, but they may directly curb prolactin production and slow down its daily secretion. In any case, chaste tree's ability to lower prolactin levels is an important effect because high prolactin levels lead to decreased progesterone. And remember that without progesterone opposing its action, estrogen is allowed to continue to build up your uterine lining unimpeded throughout the month, resulting in heavy bleeding during your period.

If you are experiencing heavy bleeding or erratic periods and want to try chaste tree berries, buy a product that's standardized to contain 0.5 percent agnuside and 0.6 percent aucubin. The recommended dosage is one 175-milligram tablet once a day. If you prefer to use a tincture, take 3 to 5 millilitres (1/2 to 1 teaspoon) once a day. There are a few herbal supplements for menopause that combine chaste tree berries with other herbs like black cohosh and dong quai. You can certainly try these, but if you don't find them effective it may be because they offer too little of each ingredient.

Chaste tree berry is not fast acting; it takes some time for it to produce results. You should plan on using it for at least four to six months. Chaste tree berry should not be combined with hormone replacement therapy and should be discontinued if you become pregnant. Side effects are rare. A few cases of gastrointestinal upset and mild skin rash have been reported. Also, be sure to let your doctor know that you are taking chaste tree berry if you're on any medication that interacts with dopamine receptors in the brain. Two common drugs that do this are the antidepressants Wellbutrin® and Effexor®, but there are other drugs that influence dopamine levels as well—ask your doctor or pharmacist. If you are taking chaste tree at the same time as these drugs, your doctor will want to monitor you closely to make sure that the herb doesn't make your medication less effective.

THE bottom LINE...

Leslie's recommendations for managing heavy menstrual flow

1   If you experience heavy flow during your periods, increase your intake of iron-rich foods. Every day, choose at least two iron-rich foods.

2   Make sure that your multivitamin and mineral supplement contains 15 to 18 milligrams of iron. A multivitamin containing this amount of iron will likely be sold as a "woman's" supplement. At menopause, when you are no longer menstruating, switch to a regular formula that contains no more than 10 milligrams of iron.

3   If heavy flow has plagued you for some time and your energy levels are down, ask your family doctor to measure your iron level.

    If iron deficiency anemia is diagnosed by your blood test, take 100 milligrams of iron two or three times a day two hours after meals. After six to eight weeks your doctor will retest your blood to determine your iron levels. Once iron supplements are discontinued, return to your multivitamin and mineral supplement. Since iron supplements can cause stomach upset and constipation they are often better tolerated when taken later in the day (afternoon and evening). Iron-only supplements should be taken *only* if your doctor has diagnosed anemia.

    Aim to consume between 25 and 35 grams of fibre per day to help prevent the constipation associated with iron supplements.

4   Consider taking a standardized extract of chaste tree berries to alleviate erratic periods or heavy menstrual flow. Take a 175-milligram dose once a day. Keep in mind that this herb does not work overnight. You should take it for at least four

to six months before making a decision as to whether it helps or not. Since heavy bleeding is a perimenopausal symptom that does eventually go away, chaste tree berry may not be a practical option for you— by the time it has an effect, your heavy bleeding may be over and done with. Do not take this herb if you're on hormone replacement therapy.

managing your weight

"Losing weight is only half the battle. The real
work is keeping it off. When I finally told myself
that everything I did to lose those 10 pounds is
everything I have to do to keep them off, I was
finally successful. I said goodbye to foolish diets
and changed my ways once and for all."

preventing weight gain

"I used to be able to just add a little exercise or cut back a little to manage my weight. Now I have to exercise at least three or four times a week and watch what I eat all the time. It's a real struggle!"

7

For many women (myself included), weight control is a major concern. Since I was a teenager I've had to watch what I eat and exercise regularly in order to maintain a healthy weight. Some women, on the other hand, find that staying trim comes naturally and they don't have to work very hard at it. But as menopause approaches, many of these same women find that for the first time in their life, it becomes more difficult to take off a few unwanted pounds. Or they complain about a "softening around the middle" despite their best efforts at weight control. Many of my clients have also found that weight gain is an annoying side effect of hormone replacement therapy. One reason is that hormone replacement therapy causes fluid retention. Yet, despite its uncomfortable side effects of bloating and fluid retention, hormone replacement may actually prevent the accumulation of body fat around the middle that's often reported by post-menopausal women.

Israeli researchers studied 63 early post-menopausal women for one year; one-half of these women took estrogen and progestin replacement therapy and the other half refused hormone therapy. At the end of 12 months, body weight and body fat had increased significantly in *both* groups. However, there was a significant shift from lower body fat to abdominal fat in the women who did not take hormones. This redistribution of body fat from the hips to the waist was not seen in the women taking hormone replacement therapy![1] It would seem that at menopause, some women see a *shift* in their weight, not necessarily an increase on the scale. Others definitely experience weight increases and difficulty keeping the extra pounds off.

perimenopausal weight gain

There are a number of reasons why women have a difficult time controlling their weight during the perimenopausal years. It's not true that menopause itself makes women gain weight. In fact, no evidence supports the notion that a deficiency of estrogen causes body fat to accumulate. However, as the Israeli study above demonstrates, hormones may affect the activity of our fat cells and influence how our fat is distributed.

What are some of the factors that do contribute to perimenopausal weight gain? We know that our metabolic rate, which determines the speed at which our body burns calories, slows with aging. I have always maintained, however, that regular workouts, consisting of aerobic exercise and weight training, can prevent much of this age-related slowdown. In fact, the most common cause of weight gain—at any age!—is inactivity. But here's something that you might not have known—a woman's metabolic rate increases during the last 14 days of her menstrual cycle (just in time to help us handle those chocolate cravings!). With menopause then, comes a loss of this cyclic increase in metabolic rate and this may account for some weight gain.

For the most part though, mid-life weight gain is a result of poor eating habits and too little exercise. The most common dietary mistakes I see women make include the following:

- Eating too much starch—bagels, pasta, bread, low fat muffins, and the like.
- Enjoying desserts and sweets too often.
- Drinking too many alcoholic beverages.
- Not eating at regular intervals throughout the day.

All of these habits will impact on your ability to manage your weight. I have helped scores of peri- and post-menopausal women lose weight, both women taking hormone replacement and those not doing so. Making smart changes with respect to *what* you eat, *how* you eat, and *how you exercise* can help you fit comfortably into your clothes once again.

CALORIES OR FAT?

I'm sure you're familiar with the notion that if you cut back on fat and don't worry about counting calories, you'll lose weight. Cutting back on fat isn't all you need to do to lose weight, but there is some truth to this idea. The foods we eat contain three basic nutrients: carbohydrate, protein, and fat. All three provide our bodies with calories. Some foods, like milk and yogurt, are made up of a combination of all three nutrients, while other foods—oils or grains for instance—are predominantly made up of one nutrient (in this case, fat and carbohydrate, respectively). One gram (less than a teaspoon) of protein gives your body four calories, one gram of carbohydrate also provides four calories, and the same amount of fat packs nine calories, more than double. That's the rationale for cutting back on fat to help oneself lose weight. Calories from fat add up quickly and reducing the amount of fat you eat can make a big impact on your calorie intake. So, at the end of the day, it still comes back to eating fewer calories. Note also that the cutting back on fat strategy will only work if you're actually eating a high fat diet; these days many of us are careful when it comes to fat.

Indeed, you've probably heard nutritionists quoted in the media, lamenting the fact that despite the fact that we are eating less fat than we did 20 years ago, we are heavier than ever. Besides not exercising enough, what are we doing wrong? It seems we are eating more carbohydrate than ever. In our state of fat phobia, whether in an effort to shed a few pounds or to lower our cholesterol, we're eating baked potato chips, fat free cookies, and muffins, bagels, and plenty of pasta with tomato sauce. We seem to think that as long as it doesn't contain fat, it's free for the taking. Well, all nutrients, be it fat, carbohydrate, or protein, have calories and if you eat too much of any of them, your body stores the excess as fat. For instance, eating that low fat bagel (it certainly seems like a better choice than a fat laden muffin) is actually the same thing, calorie-wise, as eating four or five slices of bread. When's the last time you sat down to five pieces of toast for breakfast? By the time you've finished your Italian meal of pasta and bread, you've probably had the equivalent of six (or more) slices of bread! In other words, even though your calories aren't coming from fat, they are still adding up.

dietary approaches

TODAY'S FAD DIETS

The question remains, how should you eat to successfully lose weight? Should you eat a high carbohydrate, low fat diet? Or should you try one of the high protein, low carbohydrate diets? Is there any truth to food combining? To choosing foods based on your blood type? Well, I can understand if you're confused. These days there is certainly no shortage of diet books on the market, each claiming that its own special formula is guaranteed to make those readers who diligently follow the protocols given become thin and healthy. To help you sort out the useless from the useful, I've summarized today's popular (but not necessarily sound) weight loss diets. And in Appendix 1, I'll give you my own weight loss diet plan. Now, let's take a look at some of the most popular diets on the market today.

Dr. Atkin's Diet and The Protein Power Plan

Both of these diets are high in protein, fairly high in fat, and contain almost no carbohydrate. They don't allow you to eat more than 20 to 30 grams of carbohydrate each day—the amount found in one and one-half slices of bread or one-half of a medium sized banana. These diets promote "ketosis," an abnormal metabolic state. The brain and central nervous system rely on carbohydrate as a fuel source and after two days without carbohydrate, they must adapt to a new energy source. That adaptation is called ketosis. In this state, the body breaks down fat into ketones, which are then used by the brain and central nervous system as fuel.

These diets are intended for short term use only. Studies have found that being in ketosis for a long period of time increases the risk of heart disease by damaging your low density lipoprotein (LDL) cholesterol. Once LDL cholesterol is damaged, it is more likely to stick to artery walls. You'll find more detailed information on LDL cholesterol in Chapter 9, "Reducing Your Risk of Heart Disease."

FOURTEEN FAMOUS WEIGHT LOSS BLUNDERS

1 Not exercising regularly.
2 Going on a binge the week before going on a "diet."

3 Fasting to lose weight.

4 Skipping meals in an effort to save up calories for the next.

5 Going to a salad bar and heaping on cheeses, meats, pasta mixed with mayonnaise, marinated vegetables, and salad dressing.

6 Having an "on-a-diet" or an "off-a-diet" mentality, rather than eating moderately and carefully all the time.

7 Thinking of higher calorie foods as "bad" or "forbidden," rather than as something that can be enjoyed now and then.

8 Expecting to lose more than two pounds per week.

9 Losing weight to look good for someone else.

10 Losing weight so that you can become a wonderful person—you've forgotten that you already are a wonderful person.

11 Thinking of losing weight as something you have to do, rather than as something you're choosing to do.

12 Thinking you're overweight when you're not.

13 Not giving yourself enough time to buy, prepare, or eat your meals.

14 After reaching your desired weight, not taking charge the moment you discover that your weight has crept up a few pounds.

Dr. Atkin's New Diet Revolution

This diet involves a strict 2-week "induction" (induction of ketosis) then a gradual reintroduction of carbohydrate. Most people who come off this diet gain weight quickly. That's because when you start eating carbohydrate again your body rebuilds its glycogen (carbohydrate) stores in your liver and muscles. For every gram of carbohydrate stored, you store three grams of water. The net result? Rapid weight gain. The Atkin diet is not the answer for long term weight control. It's a diet you go "on and off" of. It doesn't change your eating habits over the long-term. Furthermore, no studies have been published on the long-term success of high protein, very low carbohydrate diets.

Protein Power

Written by medical doctors Michael and Mary Eades, *Protein Power* is another plan that puts you into ketosis. The first phase of the diet allows you to eat no more than 30 grams of carbohydrate each day (the equivalent of two regular slices of bread) and lasts for four to six weeks. Then you enter the second phase when you're allowed to eat a little more carbohydrate (a whopping 55 grams a day). This level of carbohydrate intake is followed until you reach your weight and health goals. Then the maintenance phase has you gradually increase your carbohydrate intake at each meal. So once again, the *Protein Power* diet is not a diet for life. It does, however, encourage you to eat more fibre and healthier types of fat than the other protein based diet discussed above and recommends a multivitamin and daily potassium supplement. That's because the authors recognize that ketosis is a powerful diuretic and causes your body to lose fluid and minerals, especially potassium and sodium. Not replacing lost potassium can have serious health consequences. While a pill might take care of your potassium needs for a time, does this high protein approach sound like a healthy way to lose weight?

There are other health risks associated with high protein diets. In order to prevent dehydration while on these diets, you must drink plenty, and I mean plenty, of water. As just mentioned, ketosis causes your body to excrete large amounts of water, sodium, and potassium. If you choose fatty meats and cheese as your main protein foods you run the risk of high blood cholesterol levels. Your liver uses saturated fat in animal food to manufacture blood cholesterol. And because you're allowed virtually no fruit or dairy products on these diets, you won't be meeting your needs for certain nutrients, especially vitamins C, D, and folic acid, and the mineral calcium. What's more, these diets often cause constipation due to a lack of fibre.

If you take medication for high blood pressure, high cholesterol, or diabetes, and you decide to try a high protein diet, your doctor should monitor you. These diets are definitely not appropriate for people with kidney problems since high amounts of protein stress the kidneys. And if you're someone who exercises regularly, these diets won't provide fuel for your muscles. Whether you are a weight trainer, a jogger, or a tennis player, it's carbohydrate that fuels your workouts.

The Zone

The Zone describes a low carbohydrate, moderate protein, low fat diet developed by Dr. Barry Sears. The "Zone" diet does not cause ketosis because it doesn't eliminate carbohydrates (I'll give it points for this). Rather, Dr. Sears advocates eating meals and snacks that are made up of 40 percent carbohydrate, 30 percent protein, and 30 percent fat. Supposedly this combination of nutrients promotes the right balance of two hormones important in blood sugar regulation, called insulin and glucagon. If your diet encourages you to produce less insulin, says the author, your body will burn your fat stores and cause you to lose weight.

While no clinical study has proven that The Zone diet results in weight loss attributable to achieving a certain balance of hormones in your bloodstream, the plan does have a few nutritional merits. For one, the diet recommends you eat those starchy foods that are slowly converted to blood glucose. (Eating such foods results in lower insulin secretions after a meal.) And researchers are finding that the type of carbohydrate you eat just might affect your ability to lose weight.

Nutritionists are now classifying carbohydrate foods according to their ability to cause a rise in blood sugar, something referred to as a food's "glycemic index." A high glycemic index food (white bread, sugar) is converted to blood glucose quickly. A rapid rise in blood glucose causes your pancreas to secrete a large amount of insulin into your bloodstream. Insulin's job is to lower your blood sugar and store carbohydrates as glycogen, or if you've overeaten, as fat. The end result of high insulin production is that your blood sugar will drop off sooner and you'll soon feel hungry again. Foods with a low glycemic index (oatmeal, yogurt) take longer to digest and lead to a gradual, slow rise in blood glucose. You don't get a surge of insulin production and the energy from the food circulates in your bloodstream longer. Thus you don't feel hungry as quickly after eating foods with a low glycemic index.

RESEARCH FILE

Glycemic index and weight loss

You've already learned that starchy foods can impact the rate at which your pancreas releases insulin, the hormone that puts circulating blood sugar into storage. Starchy foods with a "high glycemic index" get converted to blood glucose quickly and cause an exaggerated insulin response. And the more insulin your body produces, the more sugar is removed from your blood, and the sooner you're likely to be hungry again. Indeed, researchers have found a strong link between avoidance of high glycemic foods and successful weight control.

A recent American study offered overweight teenage boys unlimited snacks for five hours after giving them meals with low (vegetable omelet and fruit), medium (regular oatmeal), or high glycemic (instant oatmeal) foods. The boys ate nearly twice as much in snacks after the high glycemic meal as compared to after the low glycemic meal. The researchers also found that the boys' blood sugar and insulin rose the highest and fastest after a high glycemic index meal, but then crashed. A crash in blood sugar, as already explained, leads to hunger and possibly, overeating.[2]

My advice? If you're going to eat a starchy meal accompanied by very little protein, choose a meal emphasizing a low glycemic food like pumpernickel bread, whole grain rye bread, legumes, barley, brown rice, yams, wholewheat pasta, All Bran cereal, Red River cereal, or Cream of Wheat.

The Zone diet also encourages the consumption of protein foods lower in fat, like chicken breast and fish, and it promotes the use of healthy fats and oils. Sounds fine so far. Are there any drawbacks to this diet? Well, I'll warn you right now that *The Zone* is a complicated book to understand and you may find the instructions highly impractical. A Zone lunch might include 3 ounces (90 grams) of lean protein, one-quarter of a pumpernickel bagel, and low glycemic index vegetables. For the most part, following this diet means bringing your meals to work or school. Many people find that the carbohydrate portions from bread, grains, fruits, and vegetables are very limiting. For instance, you might be allowed three carbohydrate servings (called blocks) at a meal. A carbohydrate serving could be one-quarter cup (50 millilitres) kidney beans, one-half apple, one-fifth cup (30 millilitres) of brown rice, or one-quarter cup (50 millilitres) of pasta. It's easy to see that you'll be eating much less carbohydrate from starchy foods and fruit. This diet also lacks calcium. A small one-half cup (125 millilitres) portion of plain yogurt or low fat milk is allowed only as a daily snack, not at meals. According to my calculations, this diet provides *at most* 500 milligrams of calcium per day. If you decide to follow it, you'll definitely need to take a supplement to reach your daily requirement of 1,000 to 1,500 milligrams.

Sugar Busters!

Sugar Busters! is by four medical doctors: H. Steward, M. Bethea, S. Andrews, and L. Balart. Like the diet given in *The Zone*, this diet is based on the concept of eating foods that minimize the amount of insulin your body secretes. The authors contend that if you produce less insulin, you won't store body fat and, even better, you'll mobilize your fat stores. This diet limits your portions of starchy foods and only carbohydrates with a low glycemic index are recommended. That means that if you follow this diet, you can't eat white bread, white rice, white pasta, watermelon, potatoes, corn, or even beets. That leaves you with brown rice, whole-grain pastas, pita bread, rye bread, high fibre cereals, sweet potatoes, legumes, most fruits, and green vegetables as better choices.

This diet does not require you to eat carbohydrate, protein, and fat in specific proportions at each meal. Starchy foods are eaten only at one or two meals daily, never at all three. On the suggested two-week meal plan, you're allowed only three servings of starch or grains each day (most balanced weight loss programs allow at least four to six servings of grain, depending on your exercise level). Although the authors do mention that portion control is important, serving sizes are not given for any of the plan's acceptable foods, not even in the 14-day meal plan.

If you're trying to lower your cholesterol level the *Sugar Busters!* plan might not be the best to follow since consumption of cheese, pâté, bacon, and plenty of red meat are encouraged. This diet has also incorporated the concept of food combining. Fruit is allowed only before or after a meal, never with a meal. The authors say that eating fruit separately leads to improved digestion, less heartburn, and less bloating. So you can forget those berries on your bowl of cereal! Calcium is another concern if you follow this diet—the daily menus provide nowhere near the recommended daily intake.

Eat Right For Your Type

This diet is based on the theory that your blood type reflects the diet and behaviour of your ancestors. The author, naturopathic physician Dr. Peter D'Adamo, says that the ancestors of Type O individuals were hunters and gatherers and therefore should eat animal protein, especially red meat. Type O people are told to limit grain and legume consumption, as these are said to encourage weight gain. The ancestors of people with Type A blood, says D'Adamo, were cultivators and supposedly do best on a vegetarian diet. They're told to limit meat, wheat, and dairy consumption. If you have type B blood then your ancestors were nomads, so you can eat a more varied diet. But corn, lentils, peanuts, sesame seeds, and wheat will apparently cause you to gain weight.

On what does Dr. D'Adamo base his advice? That's a good question. Dr. D'Adamo believes that all foods contain protein molecules called lectins, which are capable of "sticking" to the structures found on the surfaces of cells. When you eat a food that contains a lectin incompatible with your blood type, the lectins cause blood cells to clump together, usually in the vicinity of a particular organ or tissue. D'Adamo says that because of these "sticky" effects, food incompatible with your blood type can interfere with digestion, slow down your metabolism, affect insulin levels, and cause water retention. I certainly agree that the wrong foods can cause these problems in sensitive people, but until I see studies that validate this theory of how food lectins interact with blood type, it's a stretch for me to believe that such reactions have to do with blood type. Dr. D'Adamo's diet is based on observations made by his father with patients (he was a naturopathic physician too). In my view, people experience weight loss on the blood type diets because they eat tend to eat fewer calories—all of the blood type diets cut out wheat. That means no bread, pasta, bagels, crackers, cookies, or cereal. If you don't make an effort to incorporate the grain foods for your blood type, which might be rice, buckwheat, spelt, or sprouted wheat, you may very well lose weight on your blood type diet.

Fit for Life

Harvey and Marilyn Diamond were the first to popularize food combining for weight loss in the early 1980s with their book *Fit for Life: A New Way of Eating*. In a nutshell, here's the rationale behind food combining: your body uses certain enzymes to digest starch and other enzymes to break down protein. When you eat protein and starch together in the same meal, these enzymes neutralize each other and can't digest the food. So the meal ends up sitting in your stomach, rotting and forming toxins. These toxins, in turn, cause you to gain weight. On this diet then, starchy foods can only be combined with vegetables, never with protein foods like meat or chicken. Only fruit is allowed throughout the morning, and after noon it must be eaten on an empty stomach. Dairy products are forbidden, because they are a combination of protein and carbohydrate. Food combining was originally intended as a way to maximize a person's digestion and energy, and of course weight loss is an inevitable side effect for most people. Doesn't it sound like you'd be eating less food on this program? The *Fit for Life* diet is also low in calcium, and potentially deficient in protein.

I wonder what the next "breakthrough diet" will be? It seems we've come full circle. From the high protein Scarsdale and Atkin diets of the 70s to the *Protein Power* of the 90s. And food combining has resurfaced in Michel Montignac's *Eat Yourself Slim* and Suzanne Somers' *Get Skinny*. Is there any truth to all these diet prescriptions? I'm not talking about the high protein diets, which put you into ketosis (they're a whole different ball game than the other diets and I don't recommend them). But does minimizing insulin levels, combining the proper foods, or eating meals to match your blood type hold the key to long term weight control? Well, people do lose weight on these programs. But usually that's because once they start following these diets, people eat less food, plain and simple. All of these diets eliminate junk food and usually one whole food group. When you can no longer have a bagel for breakfast or a plate of pasta for dinner, you are going to eat fewer calories because you'll be eating a lot less starch (not to mention less peanut butter, cream cheese, and pesto sauce!). When you can no longer combine tuna or turkey with bread, you're going to be eating a lower calorie sandwich. With the exception of the diet outlined in *Eat Right for Your Type,* the magic of these diets lies in the fact that most of them provide about 1,200 to 1,400 calories each day. And that's a weight loss diet. They work because they force people to eat less food, period.

And many people do report feeling healthier and more energetic on these programs. When you cut back your food intake and make healthier choices you will feel better. And that's a good thing. If you do decide to give one of these diets a try (I don't mean the ketosis diets), just make sure you are making up for any missing nutrients. It might be a wise idea to consult your local dietitian for advice on what supplements you might take. If you have access to the Internet, visit the Dietitians of Canada website (www.dietitians.ca) to locate a consulting dietitian in your community.

If you're thinking about spending money on a commercial weight loss program, whether it's Weight Watchers, Jenny Craig, or a program at your local hospital, first determine if the program is right for you. The questions I've outlined in "Choosing a Program," below, will help you decide if the program is credible and if it will suit your needs.

choosing a program

Before you sign up for a weight loss program, ask yourself the following questions, and check off the ones that apply. When you're finished, take a look at how the pros and cons of the program you're interested in stack up.

Pros

- ☐ Does the program include a nutrition education component?
- ☐ Will I learn healthy eating skills?
- ☐ Does the program emphasize weight maintenance?
- ☐ Does the program promote and emphasize exercise?
- ☐ Does the program incorporate behavioural therapy and/or stress management techniques?
- ☐ Does the program address how to create social support systems that will back your attempt at weight loss?
- ☐ Are the counsellors clearly well qualified?

Cons

- ☐ Does the program exclude any one food group?
- ☐ Does the program rely on any type of meal supplement?
- ☐ Does the program rely on specially purchased foods?
- ☐ Is the same approach used for men and women?
- ☐ Do the counsellors seem not well qualified or experienced?

Your call

- ☐ Does the program offer one-on-one and/or group sessions?

LESLIE'S DIET STRATEGIES FOR WEIGHT LOSS

Before I give you my advice on how to lose weight or prevent weight gain, let me say that I don't for one minute believe that one diet, or one way of eating, is right for all people. When I develop weight loss plans for clients I ask about their food preferences, frequency of food cravings, exercise routine, past weight loss attempts, and other lifestyle issues. This information helps me determine the best type of diet for my client. In some cases, high carbohydrate/low fat works well, and in other situations a higher protein diet is a better approach. In Appendix 1, you'll find my recommended meal plan for achieving and maintaining a healthy weight. But before you decide to cut back your food intake, take a minute to assess your current weight by looking at the following section.

Do I really need to lose weight?

While being overweight can increase your risk of heart disease and breast cancer, your risk is only partially determined by the number you see on the bathroom scale. Once you complete this assessment, you'll have a more complete picture of how your weight is likely to affect your health. Don't worry, the meanings of all the calculations will be explained once you've done them!

What's your BMI?

Calculate your body mass index (BMI) as follows:

1. Divide your weight in pounds by 2.2 = weight in kilograms (kg).
2. Multiply your height in inches by 2.54 = height in centimetres (cm).
3. Divide your height (cm) by 100 = height in metres.
4. Square your height in meters (multiply the number representing your height by itself).
5. Your BMI = weight (in kg) divided by the number obtained in calculation (4) above.

Long term studies show that the overall risk of developing chronic disease is generally related to your BMI as follows:

- BMI of 20 to 25: Risk is very low; healthy range.
- BMI of 25 to 27: Your risk is starting to increase; caution zone.
- BMI over 27: Moderate risk.
- BMI 30 or more: High risk.

Waist/hip ratio

Calculate your waist/hip ratio as follows:

1. Using a tape measure, measure the circumference of your waist at its narrowest point, when your stomach is relaxed.
2. Next, measure the circumference of your hips at their widest. (Sorry girls! This is where your buttocks stick out the most.)
3. Finally, divide your waist measurement by your hip measurement.

When it comes to your waist/hip ratio, a healthy target is 0.8 or less. At this ratio, you're not carrying excess weight around your middle. It's especially fat around the abdomen that can lead to health problems. You might not appreciate hefty hips and thighs, but at least they don't increase your health risk.

You must remember that there are factors other than weight that increase your risk of disease. Poor diet, excessive alcohol consumption, a lack of exercise, smoking, and the presence of high blood pressure are other important risk factors for disease.

Is the time right?

If you've done the calculations and it seems that losing some weight would be a good idea, you need to take one more step before embarking on a weight loss program. You need to determine if this is a good time for you to make a lifestyle change. Otherwise your chances of success are slim. Think about the following questions:

- How motivated are you this time? Compare your present level of motivation to your state of mind during previous attempts to change your eating habits and exercise patterns. Is there something special about the way you're feeling now?
- Are you looking at a long-term commitment? Can you envision yourself still cooking healthy foods and working out a year from now?
- Is your life full of outside stresses? If so, now is probably not the time to start a lifestyle change.
- How much weight do you expect to lose? How quickly? Are your goals realistic?
- How do you feel about fitting exercise into your daily schedule?
- Do you have friends, family members, or coworkers who will support you in your efforts? If not, would you consider joining a support group or starting one?
- Are you easily swayed from your healthy habits by social occasions?
- Do you eat when you feel lonely, bored, anxious, or depressed? If so, do you feel ready to come up with alternative responses to these feelings?
- When you go off your plan or miss a workout, how quickly can you get back on track?
- If you binge, use laxatives or diuretics, or induce vomiting, do you have strategies for changing this behaviour by yourself? If not, would you consider seeing a therapist or eating-disorder specialist?

Strategic weight loss

If you're still reading, it's likely that the numbers say you need to lose weight—and that you feel ready to tackle the challenge. Here are some of the key strategies I encourage clients to implement so that they will successfully lose weight—and keep it off.

Set a realistic goal   Take a look at what your weight has been for the past 10 to 15 years. If you want to weigh 130 pounds, but you haven't been there since your early 20s, keep in mind that your goal might be more difficult to achieve. In fact, depending on your lifestyle today, it may be unrealistic. Also, don't think you have to rely on the scale to set a goal. I have many clients who choose a size of clothing as their target. Others prefer to measure their success by improvements in physical fitness, or improvements in blood cholesterol or blood pressure readings. If you do decide on a number on the scale, make sure you pick a five-pound weight range that you want to stay within. It's not realistic to expect yourself to remain a constant weight. You need a little room for holidays and entertaining.

Have the right mindset   Think long-term lifestyle change instead of short-term quick fix. I can tell you right now that people who approach losing weight with this attitude are far more successful. Before you embark on a weight loss program, ask yourself what your motivation is. Are you trying to fit into a dress for your son's wedding next month? Or do you want to be healthier and have more energy? The right mindset also means being comfortable with slow and steady weight loss. Any weight loss plan shouldn't cause you to lose much more than two pounds per week. When you lose weight at a faster rate, chances are good you're losing muscle and water. And the more muscle you lose, the slower the rate at which your body burns calories.

Get social support   If you need help from a spouse, family member, coworker, or friend, ask for it. It often helps to have a workout partner, especially if you're just beginning an exercise program. If your partner pulls out potato chips every night after dinner, ask that person to be mindful of your attempt to change your eating habits. If you want positive reinforcement from someone, let that person know.

Start an exercise program   If you're not already active, it's time to get moving. Exercise burns calories, and by building up muscle it helps your body to burn more calories while at rest. To help you lose body fat, aim to get four cardiovascular workouts each week (brisk walking, jogging, stair climbing, swimming, cross-country skiing, aerobics classes). Start exercising for 20 minutes per session, and gradually build up to a minimum of 30 minutes each session. When you're ready, add two or three weight training sessions per week. Studies have found that adding weight training to a weight loss program speeds up weight loss. If you're currently completely sedentary, remember to consult your doctor before starting an exercise program.

Eat at regular intervals   Eating a meal or snack every four to five hours will help to boost your metabolism, improve your energy level, and help you maintain a consistent blood sugar level. Eating regularly prevents hunger and helps to eliminate snacking or overeating at the next meal.

Don't eat dinner late   Ideally, finish eating dinner no later than eight o'clock. Remember that as the evening approaches, your body's metabolism naturally slows down. Dinnertime is actually when your body needs the smallest meal (but of course this is when most of us eat the bulk of the day's calories). If you get home late, tell yourself that you've missed dinner. Just because you walk in the door doesn't mean you have to have dinner. Have a light snack instead—some yogurt, a piece of fruit, or a bowl of soup.

Snack wisely   If any two of your day's meals will be more than five hours apart, plan to snack between them. Between-meal snacks are important to help keep your energy levels up and prevent snacking on sweets (or some other unhealthy food). Depending on the meal, your blood sugar will drop three to four hours later. Since your blood sugar is the only source of fuel for your brain, a post-meal dip can make you feel sluggish and tired. Often this is when people go in search of a "pick-me-up." So instead of letting a blood sugar low push you into rash action, plan to give yourself the needed energy boost at the right time. But here's my rule—*no snacking on starchy foods* like bagels, pretzels, low fat cookies, low fat crackers, or fat free muffins. Because these foods are quickly converted to blood glucose (remember, they're high glycemic index foods) they're more likely to lead to further hunger and sweet cravings. (For a look at the glycemic index of various foods, check out my Research File, "Choosing Low Glycemic Carbohydrates," on page 83.) Better snacks include yogurt, milk, homemade smoothies, and whole fruit which will also help you get more fibre and calcium into your diet.

NUTRITION TIP

Diet friendly foods

Feeling hungry but don't want to sabotage your healthy eating plan? Researchers at the University of Sydney have created what they call a satiety index of various foods. They tested the ability of 240 calories worth of particular foods to satisfy one's appetite. All foods were compared to white bread, which was given a satiety index rating of 100. As you'll see, 240 calories worth of some foods were only half as satisfying as white bread, while others were three times more satisfying.[3] Take a look.

Potato	323	Cookies	120
Fish	225	Bananas	118
Oatmeal	209	French fries	116
Oranges	202	Bread, white	100
Apples	197	Muesli	100
Pasta, wholewheat	188	Ice cream	96
Beef steak	176	Potato chips	91
Grapes	162	Peanuts	84
Popcorn	154	Candy bar	70
Bran cereal	151	Doughnut	68
Cheese	146	Cake	65
Crackers	127	Croissant	47

Eat enough protein   Be sure to get at least six servings of protein-rich foods each day. Not only will this allow you to meet your protein needs, but protein will also help to maintain your blood sugar levels longer. I recommend splitting your protein servings between lunch and dinner. Some people prefer to include some protein at breakfast too. See Appendix 2 for what constitutes one protein serving.

Lower your starch intake   When you have pasta, don't eat bread. If you have a meal that includes rice or potatoes, don't eat bread. Too much starch adds extra calories to your day. Even though bread on its own is low in fat, it still has calories and adds up. For example, one large bagel from the Great Canadian Bagel Company is equivalent in calories to five slices of bread! Here are a few tips that might help prevent you from overeating starchy foods:

- Say no to the bread basket in restaurants.
- When you have pasta or stir-fries, skip the bread.
- At breakfast, have cereal *or* toast, not both.
- Keep your pasta portion to one cup cooked (appetizer size).
- If you find you tend to overeat foods like pasta, rice, or potatoes, you might consider skipping the starch at dinner. Enjoy grilled fish, chicken, or lean meat with plenty of vegetables.

Eat more low glycemic carbohydrates   Low glycemic carbohydrate foods take longer to digest than high glycemic carbohydrates and lead to a gradual, slow rise in blood glucose. You don't produce a surge of insulin when you eat them (insulin takes sugar out of the bloodstream), and the energy from the food therefore lasts longer. To stay satisfied longer after a snack or meal, choose legumes, barley, brown rice, baked potatoes, whole grain rye bread, whole wheat pasta, All Bran cereal, oatmeal, cream of whole wheat or brown rice, apples, oranges, milk, and yogurt. High glycemic foods include white rice, instant rice, mashed potatoes, white bread, whole wheat bread, corn flakes, muesli, puffed rice, bananas, and raisins.

NUTRITION TIP

Choosing low glycemic carbs

Nutritionists assign carbohydrate foods a glycemic index (GI) ranking based on how quickly they increase blood sugar levels. In this system, foods are compared to bread (white or whole grain), which has a reference value of 100. In the list below, instant rice has a glycemic index ranking of 124; chickpeas of 47. That means the rice increases blood sugar more quickly than bread, whereas chickpeas boost sugar levels only half as quickly as bread.

To aid weight loss, choose more foods with lower GI values (less than 90). Remember, the faster your blood sugar rises, the more insulin your pancreas secretes, and the faster your blood sugar falls. After a steep blood sugar drop, you'll tend to have increased hunger, carbohydrate cravings, and less energy for your brain! Studies also show that eating low GI foods at two meals daily can help lower elevated blood sugar, cholesterol, and triglyceride levels!

FOOD GLYCEMIC INDEX (GI) VALUES
Breads and crackers

Rice cakes	117	Brown bread	96
Soda crackers	106	Stoned Wheat Thins	96
Bagel	103	Pita bread	88
Melba toast	100	Linseed rye bread	82
White bread	100	Pumpernickel (whole grain)	66

Grains

Rice, instant	124
Rice, brown	79
Corn	78
Bulgur	68
Rice, parboiled	64
Pasta	40 to 70
Barley	36

Potatoes

Instant	118
French fries	107
Boiled and mashed	104
New, whole	81
Baked	85
Yam	73

Cereals

Corn Flakes	119
Rice Krispies	117
Corn Bran	109
Cheerios	106
Cream of Wheat	105
Shredded Wheat	99
Oatmeal	87
Red River	70
Special K	77
All Bran Buds	67
All Bran	60

Beans

Baked beans	57
Chickpeas	47
Lima beans	46
Split peas	45
Lentils, green	42
Kidney beans	42
Soybeans	25

Fruit

Watermelon	103
Raisins	91
Papaya	83
Mango	80
Fruit cocktail	79
Banana	76
Kiwi	75
Grapes	62
Orange	62
Apple	52
Peach	51
Apricots, dried	44
Plum	34
Cherries	32

Milk products

Yogurt (with sugar added)	47
Skim milk	46
Yogurt (artificially sweetened)	20

Sweets and Sweeteners

Honey	104
Arrowroot cookies	99
Table sugar	92
Ice cream	87
Digestive cookies	84
Oatmeal cookies	81

Don't eliminate fat   You need some fat to stay healthy. Just remember to keep your intake of added fats and oils to a moderate level. Aim to get three to four fat servings each day. See Appendix 2 for what constitutes one fat serving.

Treat yourself   Treat yourself to a serving of sweets, dessert, or candy once a week. Enjoy a "real" serving of whatever you really want once a week. If sweets aren't your thing, make it French fries or chicken wings. Make this weekly treat part of the plan and don't feel guilty for enjoying it. Remember that any changes you make to lose weight have to be sustainable. Can you really see yourself giving up your special treats for good?

Avoid excess sugar   I certainly don't mind a little jam on your toast or a teaspoon of sugar in your coffee. But beverages like regular pop, fruit drinks, and fruit juice only add extra calories to your day. I'd rather you quenched your thirst with water and got your fruit servings as whole fruit. You'll cut back on calories, and you'll also boost your fibre intake.

Limit alcohol   Keep your alcohol intake to no more than seven drinks per week. I explained to you earlier that one gram of pure fat has nine calories, more than double the amount in one gram of protein or carbohydrate. Well, a gram of alcohol in beer, wine, or liquor has seven calories—they add up. Perhaps even more important, I also find that alcohol consumption tends to lower one's willpower, making it more difficult to stick to a healthy meal plan. If you do drink alcohol, one drink per day is not considered to increase your risk of disease. If you're out for an evening, try sticking to one alcoholic drink and rounding out your evening with a low calorie alcohol-free beverage (mineral water, club soda, Clamato juice, cranberry and soda). One drink is equivalent to six ounces (175 millilitres) of wine, one bottle (375 millilitres) of light beer or 1.5 ounces (45 millilitres) of liquor.

Deal with lapses   We're all human. That means our weight is not intended to always measure one certain number on the scale. When you have a busy social calendar or you're spending three wonderful weeks enjoying the wine and food of Italy, you're bound to put on a few pounds. The key to long term weight maintenance is nipping small weight gains in the bud. That's why I advised you earlier to choose a *weight range* to stay within. If you want to stay trim, you've got to catch that five pound gain before it becomes ten. And if you're not watching things carefully, that 10 pounds can quite easily turn into 20. I'm sure many of you know just what I mean. I recommend monitoring your weight on a regular, weekly basis. When you see a few pounds creep on, have a plan of action to take them off. You might decide to keep a food diary for a few weeks. When you have to write down all the foods you eat, you're more likely to make healthy choices. And keeping a daily record of the food you eat gives you focus and serves as a reminder of your goals. Or you might add an extra workout to your week for a month. Some people give up sweets until the pounds are back down. Do whatever will work for you.

WEIGHT MANAGEMENT

Listed below are the major behaviours associated with successful weight control. Place a check next to those behaviours that are a regular part of your life. Then comes the hard part. Take a look at the behaviours that aren't yet part of your daily routine. Choose one and begin practising it until it is. Then choose another behaviour you're currently not practising and do the same thing until every behaviour on this list is part of your life!

☐ I maintain a positive, optimistic attitude about my ability to control my weight.

☐ I set small, bite-sized goals on the way to my weight target.

☐ I keep a food and activity record, so I always know how well I'm doing and why my weight is fluctuating the way it is.

☐ I recognize and reward my successes.

☐ I monitor my weight by how my clothes fit, not only by what the scale reads.

☐ I make healthy eating choices that are consistent with my lifestyle needs.

☐ I select low fat milk and milk products.

☐ I eat breakfast regularly.

☐ I go no longer than five hours at a time without eating.

☐ I spend at least 20 minutes eating each meal.

☐ I stop eating when I feel satisfied, not when I'm full.

☐ I stay aware of the portion sizes I am eating.

☐ I enjoy eating meals with family and friends.

☐ I recognize when I eat for reasons other than hunger.

☐ I reserve high fat or sweet treats for special occasions, rather than vowing never to eat them again.

☐ I include a variety of physical activities in my lifestyle.

vitamins and minerals

MULTIVITAMIN AND MINERAL SUPPLEMENTS

Should you take a "multi" if you're on a lower calorie diet? I say yes. If you are following a low calorie diet (less than 1,500 calories daily) you'll likely experience a shortfall of vitamins and minerals. Even when you aren't cutting back on calories, it is a challenge to meet your requirements for certain nutrients important in longterm health. For instance, each day women need 400 micrograms of folate (folic acid), a B vitamin that plays a role in protecting us from heart disease. To get the minimum 400 micrograms, you'd have to make sure you eat plenty of whole grains, and a serving of spinach, lentils, or orange juice on a daily basis. A low calorie diet also presents a challenge as far as meeting your iron requirements is concerned. And if you're over 50, you need to get vitamin B12 from a supplement or from fortified foods. That's because as we get older, our stomachs produce less hydrochloric acid, making it more difficult to absorb B12 from our foods.

So you can see that a multivitamin and mineral supplement offers you a little extra nutritional insurance. A good one will provide you with the recommended daily amounts of all the key vitamins and minerals, except for your daily rations of calcium, vitamin E, and possibly iron. Here's what you should look for when choosing a product:

- When it comes to iron, premenopausal women should buy a supplement containing at least 10 milligrams of iron, preferably 15 milligrams. Post-menopausal women have lower iron requirements and can choose a multi containing 10 milligrams or less.
- Look for a supplement that offers 0.4 to 1.0 milligrams of folic acid.
- A multivitamin/mineral should contain beta carotene, vitamin A, and vitamins D, B1, B2, B6, B12, and folic acid. Biotin and pantothenic acid aren't important since they're easily supplied by food.
- In terms of minerals, a supplement should contain iron, copper, zinc, magnesium, iodine, selenium, and chromium. Don't worry if you don't see phosphorus or potassium since these minerals are widely available in food.
- Take your supplement with food to allow for better breakdown and absorption of the pill. Plan to take your supplement at the meal you are most likely to remember it. For me it's breakfast, the meal I am always home for unless I travel. And if I do travel, I put my vitamins in a special pill container I bought at the

drug store. Actually, I fill this container once a week and use it every day. It saves me the hassle of opening up a number of bottles every morning. Those other bottles, of course, contain vitamin E and calcium.

- Don't pay much attention to such terms as "natural," or "slow release."(Remember, though, that you should seek out "natural source" vitamin E.) Don't be impressed by the addition of amino acids, ginseng, or other herbs. Some multivitamins contain small amounts of protein, other nutrients, or herbs. The tiny dosage you'll receive from a multivitamin supplement won't add any benefit to your body, however. (The main purpose of such additions is probably to add market appeal to the product.)

IRON

You've already heard me say that if you're following a low calorie diet, chances are you're not getting enough iron. If you are still getting a period you need 13 milligrams of iron each day; if you've hit menopause, 9 milligrams daily is sufficient. A daily multivitamin and mineral pill will help you meet your needs. But also make an effort to boost the iron content of your diet. See page 46 for a list of foods rich in iron.

Only iron found in animal foods (called heme iron) is well absorbed by your body. That's why red meat is such a good source. Not only does it pack a fair amount of the mineral, but what it contains is also well absorbed. Ironically, the iron-rich foods we eat the most of—whole grains, beans, dried fruit, and vegetables—offer a less available form of iron (called non-heme iron). If this is the first chapter of this book you've read, I'll bet you didn't know that if you have a source of vitamin C with plant foods rich in iron, your body will absorb up to four times more of the iron! So here are a few iron boosting combinations:

- Whole grain cereal with strawberries.
- Stoneground toast with orange juice.
- Cream of Wheat cereal with dried cranberries.
- Whole wheat waffles topped with kiwi slices and blueberries.
- Spinach salad with orange segments.
- Broccoli and red pepper stir-fry with brown rice.
- Whole wheat spaghetti with rapini and olive oil.
- Brown beans in tomato sauce.

Here are a few other tips that will help you enhance your body's absorption of non-heme iron:

- Include a little animal protein with your meal. The presence of heme iron in a meal will enhance the absorption of the non-heme iron eaten at that same meal. It only takes a few ounces of meat, fish, or eggs to achieve this effect.
- Don't drink coffee or tea with meals rich in iron. The tannins in these beverages interfere with iron absorption. Drink coffee or tea one hour before or one hour after a meal.
- Foods high in calcium and phosphorus (dairy products) can slightly inhibit iron absorption. Don't combine foods rich in iron with large quantities of milk or yogurt.

CALCIUM

Here's another example of an important mineral that's often missing in a diet designed for weight loss. The even sadder truth is that this bone building mineral is often lacking in high calorie diets too. You'll read all about calcium in Chapter 8, but I do want to make sure you know how to make up for what you might be missing.

To start, you do need to know that most of you need 1,000 milligrams of calcium each day, and if you're over 50, you should be aiming for 1,200 milligrams. If you are at risk for osteoporosis, or you have the disease, then 1,500 milligrams daily is a must. Here are a few of the top calcium sources in the average diet:

CALCIUM CONTENT OF COMMON FOODS (MILLIGRAMS)

Milk, 1 cup (250 ml)	300
Milk, calcium enriched, 1 cup (250 ml)	420
Yogurt, plain, 3/4 cup (175 ml)	300
Yogurt, fruit flavoured, 3/4 cup (175 ml)	250
Cheese, hard 1.5 ounces (45 g)	300
Fortified soy or rice beverage, 1 cup (250 ml)	300
Calcium fortified orange juice, 1 cup (250 ml)	300
Tofu, raw firm (with calcium sulphate), 4 oz. (120 g)	260
Blackstrap molasses, 2 tbsp. (25 ml)	288
Bok choy, cooked, 1 cup (250 ml)	158

Swiss chard, cooked, 1 cup (250 ml)	102
Broccoli, cooked, 1 cup (250 ml)	94

For every 300 milligrams of your daily calcium target missing from your diet, take a 300 milligram calcium citrate supplement with magnesium (2:1 ratio) and vitamin D added. Calcium citrate is much more easily absorbed than calcium carbonate. Calcium carbonate requires a lot of stomach acid to be well absorbed. If you take acid blocking medication for ulcers or heartburn, don't give the carbonate form a second thought. Calcium citrate is your best bet. If you need to take more than one calcium pill (most calcium citrate supplements don't come any larger than 350 milligrams of calcium per pill), split your dose over two or three meals. For those of you who don't like to swallow pills, there are some chewable calcium citrate supplements on the market.

CHROMIUM

You may have heard that this trace mineral helps burn fat and build muscle, certainly a winning combination if you're trying to lose weight. While a few studies have found that chromium supplements aided weight loss in people who exercise, most found chromium to have no effect.[4] But that doesn't mean you shouldn't worry about chromium. This mineral works hand in hand with insulin, the hormone that helps regulate your blood sugar level and your body's energy stores. With adequate amounts of chromium present, your body uses less insulin to do its job. A deficiency of chromium causes impaired blood sugar balance, increased levels of potentially harmful blood fats and cholesterol, and decreased levels of high density lipoproteins (HDLS), a desirable form of cholesterol. And if you go to the gym a lot, you might want to know that heavy exercise causes chromium to be excreted from the body.

RESEARCH FILE

Chromium and weight loss

If you've been to your health food store looking for a supplement to help you lose weight, chances are you've come across chromium. It seems there may be some truth to the claims made for chromium. While three studies have found chromium to have no effect on body weight, a few studies do point to chromium's ability to change body composition.

One large study measured the effect of chromium supplementation (200 micrograms daily) in 123 obese men and women. Study participants were assigned to either a diet/exercise/supplement combination protocol, or a diet and exercise protocol only. All participants ate 1,500 calories a day and went for five brisk 45-minute walks each week. At the end of four weeks, while there was no difference in body weight between the two groups, there was a significant difference in body composition. Those individuals taking the supplement lost more body fat and gained more muscle mass.

Another recent study found that overweight women who exercised and took 400 micrograms of chromium lost significant weight and lowered the amount of insulin their body produced in response to a carbohydrate meal. Interestingly, non-exercising women who took the same amount of chromium showed significant weight gain. This study suggests that chromium supplementation may help improve body composition (increasing the ratio of muscle to fat) when combined with regular exercise.[5]

While there's no official recommended daily intake for chromium, experts estimate that 50 to 200 micrograms per day is a safe and healthy amount to consume. Good food sources include apples with the skin, green peas, chicken breast, refried beans, mushrooms, oysters, wheat germ, and brewer's yeast. Processed foods and refined starchy foods like white bread, white rice, white pasta, sugar, and sweets all contain very little chromium. So if you're a runner who loads up on white bagels, regular pasta, and white rice, you're probably falling short of meeting your chromium needs. If you're concerned that you're not getting enough through food, check your multivitamin/mineral to see how much it contains. If it's less than 50 micrograms, you can always consider taking a separate 200 microgram supplement each day. Chromium supplements are extremely safe.

herbal remedies

Herbal remedies meant to encourage weight loss are fast becoming popular items in supplement stores. These products are generally touted to boost the consumer's metabolic rate, and thus the speed at which calories are burned. Most herbal formulas contain a few different herbs combined with other nutrients. Will these products help you lose weight? Well, that remains to be seen. No clinical studies have evaluated their long-term success. But there are some studies supporting the use of many of the individual ingredients added to a formula. I view these products as something that *might* assist you in your weight loss effort. They certainly can't take the place of a healthy diet and regular exercise. If do want to try a herbal combination to help you increase your metabolism, you need to know what's safe and what's not. Here's a look at the more popular ingredients added to products.

EPHEDRA, OR MA HUANG

Over the past few years, Ephedra (*Ephedra sinica*) has received a lot of bad press. In the United States, there have been more than 800 reported adverse reactions and 22 deaths due to ephedra abuse. The plant contains an active ingredient called ephedrine, which stimulates the central nervous system, speeds the heart rate, and increases blood pressure. When combined with other stimulant ingredients (e.g. caffeine), it increases the metabolic rate. However, taking ephedra in high doses with plenty of other stimulants does cause serious side effects. In Canada, the herb may be sold only in products that contain a combination of herbs. The law also states that the recommended dosage of such products may not give you more than 11 milligrams of ephedra daily. Even though this dose is considered safe, it can cause insomnia and anxiety in some individuals. Ephedra dependency can also occur. Because of its negative side effects, some companies have reformulated their weight loss products and removed ephedra. It seems there are safer ways to incite a metabolic boost.

BITTER ORANGE

Avantra Z™ is the latest "thermogenic" to hit the herbal supplement market. It is a patented extract made from the dried fruit of *Citrus aurantium*, also known as bitter orange (or Seville orange). It is touted to burn fat, enhance physical performance, and increase muscle, and apparently works as effectively as ephedra without any negative effects on the heart or nervous system. The herb stimulates the body's beta-3 receptors, which, in turn, elicit the breakdown of fat and catalyze an increase in the body's metabolic rate.

To explain in more detail, every cell in the body has receptor sites called alpha-1, alpha-2, beta-1, beta-2, and beta-3. The hormones we naturally produce to counter stress, adrenaline and noradrenaline, interact with these receptors to elicit a response. When these hormones interact with beta-3 receptors, fat breakdown in the body is promoted and the resting metabolic rate is increased. (Ephedra has a wider range of action than Avantra Z™ because it affects both the alpha and beta receptors. It is its impact on the alpha receptors that can cause side effects.)

Sounds good so far, but does Avantra Z™ work? A 1999 study evaluated the combined effect of bitter orange, caffeine, and St. John's Wort on weight loss in 20 overweight adults. All individuals exercised three times per week and ate an 1,800 calorie diet. At the end of a six-week period, the group receiving the herbal supplement had lost significantly more weight and body fat than the group on placebo. The combination of substances given in the study did not affect heart rate and blood pressure.[6] So it appears that bitter orange just might speed weight loss when used in conjunction with diet and exercise. You'll find the standardized extract of *Citrus aurantium* (Avantra Z™) in a few products including Quest Vitamin's TrimFit, TWINLAB's Diet Fuel® and Interactive Nutrition's Metabolean (all three products mentioned above contain a little caffeine. TrimFit and Diet Fuel also contain St. John's Wort.

HYDROXYCITRIC ACID

Here's yet another ingredient you'll find in certain weight loss formulas. Hydroxycitric acid (HCA) is an active compound found in the herb *Garcinia cambogia.* You'll find HCA sold as "Citrimax" in weight loss products. In the lab, HCA acts by inhibiting the action of a cellular enzyme and thereby increasing the breakdown of fat. But just because HCA does this in a test tube doesn't mean it works the same way in the body. I could find only two published studies that evaluated this herb in humans. Both were well controlled and found that people who took HCA burned body fat no differently than individuals taking the placebo. The larger of the two studies measured weight and fat loss in 135 overweight men and women who took either 1,500 milligrams of HCA or placebo. Both groups exercised and followed a high fibre, low calorie diet. After 12 weeks there was no significant difference between the two groups. HCA or not, both lost a significant amount of weight.[7] From what I've seen to date, there's no good evidence that HCA assists weight loss—another reason to stick to your diet and exercise routine!

WHAT'S ALL THE FUSS OVER CELLASENE™?

This herbal product found it way into the headlines in the spring of 1999 when it made its debut in North America. Developed by an Italian scientist, Cellasene™ is advertised as the breakthrough "cure" for cellulite. It is supposed to work by repairing tissues and tiny blood vessels in connective tissue found under the thighs. But other press releases that have come across my desk say Cellasene™ works by increasing blood flow, stimulating fat burning, and reducing the buildup of toxins in the body. Frankly, I'm still a little confused as to how this potion really works to get rid of cellulite. Unfortunately, there's no evidence to back the product's claims. One small, poorly controlled study has been done; it has been heavily criticized. There's also limited data available to evaluate this product's safety. And at the time of writing this book, the company that makes Cellasene™ is being investigated by the United States Food and Drug Administration for making unsubstantiated claims.

Cellasene™ is made of a combination of gingko biloba, sweet clover, bioflavonoids, dried fucus extract (a sea vegetable), evening primrose oil, and grape seed extract. Considered individually, these ingredients do have positive effects on circulation and blood vessel health. Whether they get rid of cellulite once taken in combination is an open question—at the time of writing this book, not one of the ingredients in this product had been studied in relation to cellulite metabolism. But here's the catch. The manufacturer recommends that you take two to three capsules every day for eight weeks. Then you can lower your dose to one capsule per day to maintain the effect. Well, if you consider that a box of 40 capsules costs $60, you're out of pocket $250 for the first eight weeks alone! If I were you, I'd put your money into a gym membership or a few cookbooks focussing on healthy menus.

THE Bottom LINE...

Leslie's recommendations for managing your weight

1   Stay away from fad diets. Any diet that excludes one or more food groups or relies on specially purchased foods or supplements is not healthy. Nor will it teach you how to implement the long-term behavioural changes needed for ongoing weight control.

2   Consult a registered dietitian for advice.

3   Follow my meal plan for weight loss, outlined in Appendix 1.

4   If you're cutting back on calories, take a multivitamin and mineral supplement every day. Low calorie diets often don't provide enough iron, calcium, or B vitamins.

5   You need 1,000 to 1,500 milligrams of elemental calcium each day. For every 300 milligrams missing from your diet, take 300 milligrams of elemental calcium in citrate or chelate form with vitamin D added.

6   To help you meet your iron requirements, add two iron-rich foods to your diet each day.

7   If you have problems keeping your blood sugar levels stable and your diet lacks the mineral chromium, you might consider taking a 200-microgram chromium supplement. But check how much chromium is found in your multivitamin and mineral supplement first. That amount, combined with what's available in your diet, might be all you need.

8   If you've decided to take an herbal supplement to help you lose weight, choose one containing Avantra Z™. This standardized extract of *Citrus aurantium* (bitter orange), has been shown to increase the metabolic rate when combined with a little caffeine, without the side effects of ephedra. I advise you avoid products that contain ephedra (Ma huang).

9   Be sure to include exercise. Gradually build up to four cardiovascular workouts each week, 30–45 minutes in duration. Consider adding a weight training component two or three times a week. To get started, consult a certified personal trainer.

protecting your long-term health

"Why is it that we don't think about these things in our 20s and 30s? At the age of 48, I am finally taking my present and future health very seriously by eating healthy and exercising almost daily. I'm sure I should have taken more calcium and eaten less fat when I was younger. Now that I know more, I'm encouraging my daughter to start paying attention now, not later."

reducing **your risk** of osteoporosis

"All my life I have never had a problem drinking plenty of milk. That's why I was shocked when my first bone density test showed bone loss. I've always been told that when it comes to preventing osteoporosis, calcium is what matters. I guess there's more to it than that."

8

It's not uncommon to think that fragile, brittle bones are an inevitable part of the mid-life change. In fact, osteoporosis is often viewed as a natural result of menopause. But the truth is that only 25 percent of women get osteoporosis. And as you'll come to understand as you read this chapter, just because your bone density test score is low doesn't mean you'll end up with fractured bones or a hunched posture. Now don't get me wrong. I certainly don't mean to trivialize this debilitating condition. It is true that 1.4 million Canadians have osteoporosis and that the rate at which bone fractures occur among Canadians is increasing faster than ever before. What's more, the fact that we're an aging population doesn't account for our higher rate of fractured bones. It seems there's something else at play here. What I am really trying to emphasize here is that while menopause is a natural part of aging, osteoporosis is not. And if you begin taking preventive measures right now, you can lower your odds of getting this painful bone disease.

osteoporosis defined

Osteoporosis is usually a silent disease until a fracture occurs. It's characterized by low bone mass and deterioration of existing bone tissue. The thinning and deterioration of bones that occurs in osteoporosis means that they become more fragile and the risk of fracture increases. In other words, if your bones are weaker they're more likely to break. Studies do tell us that the lower the bone mass a woman (or man) has, the higher her risk of fracture. You've probably noticed that this definition of osteoporosis emphasizes *fracture risk*, not only low bone density. By the age of 50, the average Caucasian woman has a 40 percent chance of suffering at least one fracture caused by brittle bones.

While many bone fractures are not life threatening, consider this: the risk of getting a fracture is at least five times the risk of developing breast cancer. And the impact that fractures have on health is often not fully appreciated. Did you know that having a hip fracture increases the risk of dying by 16 percent? Or that close to half of elderly women who fracture their hips lose their ability to live independently? I told you earlier than not every woman ends up with osteoporosis. Nor does every woman with low bone density end up with bone fractures. To help you better understand the factors that shape your risk for osteoporosis and subsequent bone fracture, we need to take a look at bones themselves.

PEAK BONE MASS

Your bones grow in length and density until you finish your growth spurt in your teens (sometime between the ages of 11 and 14 years for girls). After the growth spurt, your bones continue to increase in density but at a slower rate. Then, sometime in your 20s, your bones achieve what's called their *peak mass* and once this occurs, they stop increasing in density. This happens any time between the ages of 20 and 30. Some experts say that our bones may even continue to build density up until the age of 35. In any case, when you reach your peak bone mass, you have the densest bone you're ever going to have. Think of peak bone mass as the maximum bone density that you are physically able to develop. An individual's peak mass is pretty much determined by genetics, but nutrition and other lifestyle factors (like type and frequency of exercise) determine whether or not you achieve your body's genetically programmed peak bone mass.

After you achieve your peak bone mass, natural bone loss begins. Before menopause, women lose bone at a rate of one percent per year, the same rate at which men lose bone. Within the first five years after menopause, women lose bone two to six times faster than premenopausal women do. By about 10 years after menopause, the rate of bone loss returns to one percent per year. During the 10-year period of rapid bone loss following menopause, some women have the potential to lose bone very quickly. Others are slow bone losers and won't lose as much bone mass.

BONE BUILDING

Despite its "dead" appearance, bone is very active tissue. Two important types of cells keep it that way. Osteoclasts break down bone. For example, osteoclasts go to work when your diet lacks calcium. Calcium is vital to all cells, not just bone cells. When there's not enough calcium available to maintain important body functions, the osteoclasts break down bone cells to release calcium into the blood. Osteoblasts, on the other hand, are responsible for building bone. These cells secrete a collagen protein compound that provides the support matrix for the bones. The collagen matrix is then filled in with bone mineral also secreted by the osteoblasts. When this bone mineral matures, it's referred to as hydroxyapatite—a cement-like substance that gives the bones their hardness and strength. Calcium is the chief ingredient of hydroxyapatite.

The osteoclasts and osteoblasts constantly remodel your bones, breaking them down cell by cell, and then rebuilding them. This is how bone density is increased in response to weight bearing exercise, like brisk walking. The physical pounding of bones stimulates osteoblasts to rebuild bone in a particular area. But before new bone can be built, some old bone must be broken down by the osteoclasts. During childhood and adolescence, osteoblast (building) activity exceeds osteoclast (breakdown) activity. In young adults up to 30 percent of the skeleton is rebuilt every year. More bone is added to areas put under stress. For example, a right-handed golfer or tennis player will have greater bone mass in their right arm than in their left. After you've achieved your peak bone mass in your 20s or 30s, osteoclast (breakdown) activity wins out.

HORMONES AND BONE HEALTH

Many different hormones influence whether bones are being broken down or rebuilt at any given time. The three main players in calcium and bone metabolism are parathyroid hormone, vitamin D, and calcitonin. It's important that you know how these hormones affect your bones because, as you'll see later, your diet can affect their actions.

Parathyroid hormone (PTH)

PTH is secreted by your parathyroid gland (you probably already figured that out) and its job is to keep your blood calcium levels stable. Because calcium is critical for blood clotting, muscle contraction, and the transmission of nerve impulses, a constant amount of the mineral must be circulated throughout your body at all times. When blood calcium falls too low (because you're not consuming enough in your diet), PTH tells your kidneys to stop excreting calcium. PTH also activates vitamin D in your body, and vitamin D, in turn, causes your intestines to absorb more dietary calcium. Finally, PTH instructs your osteoclasts (the cells that break down bone) to release calcium from your bones into your bloodstream. The net result? Your blood calcium rises to normal at the expense of bone loss. Now you see why getting plenty of calcium and vitamin D in your diet is so important for strong bones (more on that subject later).

Calcitonin

Your thyroid gland secretes calcitonin in response to a high calcium level in the bloodstream. This hormone lowers calcium to a normal level by inhibiting the action of the osteoclasts and stimulating the osteoblasts to build new bone. However, calcitonin levels decline with age and at menopause.

A number of other hormones and drugs with hormonal effects also influence the bones.

Thyroid hormone

Too much thyroid hormone from an overactive thyroid gland (hyperthyroidism) causes a higher rate of bone breakdown. I have many clients with an underactive thyroid (hypothyroidism) who take thyroid medication. If you take levothyroxin (Synthroid) it is important to have your doctor check your thyroid hormone levels regularly. If they are too high, you'll need to adjust your medication. Keeping your thyroid hormone dose in check is an important way to prevent accelerated bone loss.

Steroid drugs

Doctors use steroid drugs such as glucocorticoids (e.g. prednisone) to treat inflammatory conditions like rheumatoid arthritis, lupus, and colitis. These drugs unfortunately increase the rate of bone loss, because one of their side effects is their ability to enhance the action of PTH. If you think back to how PTH works, you'll realize that that means your bones will mobilize more calcium into your bloodstream. Anyone who takes this type of medication must be sure they're getting plenty of calcium and vitamin D.

Estrogen

Estrogen acts to protect bones. This hormone seems to be able to prevent osteoclasts from releasing calcium from the bone into the bloodstream. Estrogen also causes calcitonin and vitamin D to be released, stimulating new bone growth to occur. In other words, your premenopausal estrogen level helps vitamin D efficiently perform its jobs of increasing calcium absorption in your intestine and preventing excess calcium loss through your kidneys.

risk factors for osteoporosis

You may already have some idea of what can increase your risk for osteoporosis. Very simply put, the strength of your bones is determined by their density, their rate of healing, and the integrity of their support structures (collagen proteins). Any factor that jeopardizes your bones' density, integrity, or ability to heal themselves can increase the odds of getting osteoporosis. Here's a list of known factors that put your bones at risk:

- older age
- low bone density
- being female
- slender or petite body structure (slender people have less bone to start with than do heavier-set people)
- deficiency of estrogen (early menopause further increases the risk)
- low calcium and vitamin D intake
- cigarette smoking
- excessive alcohol intake
- excessive caffeine intake
- sedentary lifestyle
- use of certain medications (see discussion above)
- prolonged immobilization (bones need to work against the pull of gravity to maintain their density)

- family history of maternal hip fracture
- previous bone fracture of any type after the age of 50
- certain health conditions (kidney failure, hyperthyroidism, poor digestion or absorption)

RESEARCH FILE

Smoking and osteoporosis

Many studies have shown that cigarette smoking reduces bone density and increases the risk of fracture. The U.S. Nurses' Health Study revealed that women who smoked 25 or more cigarettes a day had a 60 percent higher risk of hip fracture than women who never smoked. Two other American studies reported cigarette smoking to significantly decrease bone density in the hip and lower spine of older women (and men).[1]

Smoking affects bone health by causing increased production of inactive estrogens, leading to estrogen deficiency. Studies find that women who smoke have early natural menopause, and an increased risk of bone fractures.

If you currently smoke and would like to quit once and for all, look for a smoking cessation program in your community. A good program will offer group support, stress management techniques, and strategies to help prevent relapse.

measuring bone density

Your overall risk for osteoporosis will depend on how much bone you currently have, how strong that bone is, and how fast you're losing it. The only way doctors can get a sense of what's happening in your skeleton is by taking repeated measures of your bone density. Today, the best tool available to determine your bone density is called dual-energy-X-ray absorptiometry (DEXA). The machine that creates DEXA readings uses an X-ray tube attached to a computer to measure bone density in the lower spine and the hip, two places where fractures are likely to occur. DEXA is very accurate. The test can detect a change in bone density of as little as one percent. What this test can't do, however, is detect bone fractures. And it doesn't measure bone density in the upper spine, where a series of small fractures can result in shrinking and "dowager's hump," the characteristic hunching of the spine seen in osteoporosis. Doctors use X-rays to detect these types of fractures in your upper spine.

The DEXA test is simple, fast, and absolutely painless. A complete scan can take as little as 10 minutes. You don't even have to undress. To have your lower spine or hip scanned, you'll lie comfortably on your back on a flat padded table. And you don't have to worry about fasting before your test. Since food doesn't interfere with the test results, you can eat right before you go. But you shouldn't take a calcium supplement right before since an undigested pill can be measured as part of your bone density. This can happen because when you're lying down on your back, your intestines lie on top of your spine. So skip your calcium pill on the day you're having a bone density test.

INTERPRETING TEST RESULTS

To help you understand your test results, you'll see below the results of a DEXA bone density scan done for Nancy (not her real name), a 58-year-old woman. The test begins when a computer-generated image of four vertebrae in Nancy's lumbar, or lower, spine (L1, L2, L3, and L4) is created. The computer then calculates how much bone mineral is present in each vertebra and calculates an average bone mineral density (BMD) for three vertebrae. The more densely packed bone mineral crystals are, the stronger the bone. In Nancy's report, you can see that the average density is calculated from the bone densities of L2, L3, and L4. The average density is represented visually in the graph and in the last row of the chart; in both places these three vertebrae are called L2–L4. Nancy's BMD for L2–L4 is 0.944 grams per squared centimeter (g/cm^2). You're probably wondering what this number means. Is it good or bad?

AP SPINE BONE DENSITY RESULTS

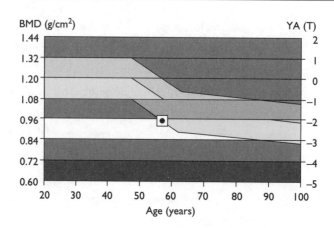

REGION	BMD (G/CM^2)	Young-Adult (%)	(T)	Age-Matched (%)	(Z)
L1	0.868	77	-2.2	86	-1.2
L2	0.969	81	-1.9	90	-0.9
L3	1.039	87	-1.3	96	-0.3
L4	0.840	70	-3.0	78	-2.0
L2-L4	0.944	79	-2.1	88	-1.1

Luckily you don't have to depend on this number alone to understand your test results. On the DEXA report, your bone density is compared to the bone density of a healthy 30 year-old woman. You can see these results under the "Young-Adult" column in the chart. In Nancy's case, the Young-Adult comparison for her lower spine (L2–L4) is 79 percent. That means Nancy's bone density is 79 percent of the average 30-year-old woman's density. In other words, she has lost 21 percent of her bone density. Every 10 percent loss of bone density, as measured against the benchmark set by a 30-year-old woman, doubles the risk of bone fracture.

Bone density results are also presented in the form of "T" scores. The T score shows the number of levels (standard deviations) between your bone density and that of a healthy 30-year-old woman. If you score one level away (one standard deviation), you are considered to have *osteopenia,* or decreased bone mass. If your test comes back saying that your bone density is more than 2.5 levels away from the healthy standard, you have *osteoporosis.* If your score is higher still and you have one or more tiny fractures, then you are considered to have *severe osteoporosis.* In Nancy's case, her T score is 2.1, which would classify her as osteopenic. How do these results influence your risk for bone fracture? Well, if you're over 65 years old, osteopenia doubles your risk for fracture, osteoporosis quadruples it, and severe osteoporosis increases the risk of bone fracture twentyfold.

You'll also notice that Nancy's DEXA results include something called an "Age-Matched" comparison. This means that Nancy's results have been compared to what is expected for women of her age. Nancy's age matched comparison is 88 percent. That means her bone density is 88 percent of what is expected for a woman her age. If your age matched comparison were unusually low, your doctor would endeavour to determine what is causing such severe bone loss.

SHOULD YOU HAVE A BONE DENSITY TEST?

If you have not yet had a DEXA test, you may be thinking that it's time you had your bone density measured. If you fall into any of the categories listed below, I recommend that you have a chat with your doctor about getting this test:

- You're approaching menopause and deciding whether to take hormone replacement therapy (HRT). The fact that HRT protects your bones is an accepted and uncontroversial medical fact. A bone density test can help you decide whether or not HRT is needed to prevent osteoporosis.
- You have a family history of osteoporosis or multiple bone fractures.
- You have premature menopause (younger than 45).
- You've been on corticosteroid drugs (e.g. prednisone) for a medical condition for three months or longer.
- You've experienced one or more episodes of longstanding malnutrition or malabsorption (for example, you have a history of anorexia nervosa, celiac disease, or Crohn's disease).
- You have a low body weight. Your body mass index (BMI) is less than 20 or you weigh less than 125 pounds (57 kg). To calculate your BMI, refer to page 78.
- You have hyperthyroidism.

Your first bone density test serves as the baseline to which future test results will be compared. If at the age of 50 your first bone density test comes back low (osteopenia) you're not necessarily heading for osteoporosis. It may be that you're a "slow loser" and later tests will find that your bone mineral content hasn't changed very much. This brings up an important point: bone density tests must be repeated every two years, to establish what your actual bone loss trends are. If future tests show that your bone density has declined rapidly between tests, your doctor will likely recommend drug treatment to slow the rate of bone loss. Here's a brief look at your options.

drug-based osteoporosis treatments

ESTROGEN THERAPY

There is no doubt in the medical and scientific community that estrogen replacement therapy reduces post-menopausal bone loss and reduces the risk of fractures. An enormous number of studies have shown that hormone replacement therapy protects the bones. Back in the 1980s the famous Framington Heart Study reported that among 3,000 Boston women, those who took estrogen when post-menopausal had a 35 percent lower risk of hip fracture as compared to those who never took hormones. Both estrogen pills and estrogen patches have been found to decrease bone loss, reduce fractures, and prevent height loss. Studies show that estrogen replacement prevents bone loss at any point in time that a woman starts to take it.[2] However, we do know that the longer a woman waits after menopause to begin HRT, the higher the chance she will lose some bone permanently. We also know that once a woman stops taking estrogen, bone loss occurs—estrogen's protective effects last only as long as a woman decides to take it. More recently, scientists have learned that a lower dose of estrogen in combination with calcium and vitamin D supplementation has a bone-conserving effect.

RESEARCH FILE

Calcium and vitamin D boost estrogen's bone building ability

Although hormone replacement therapy is currently the mainstay of osteoporosis prevention, it's often poorly tolerated because of side effects (breast tenderness, mood swings, spotting). In addition, there are health risks associated with higher doses. Scientists are now determining whether a lower dose of estrogen is able to preserve bone density in women as effectively as the higher doses that are commonly used.

Researchers at the Osteoporosis Research Center at Creighton University in Omaha, Nebraska seem to think so. In their study, 128 women over 65 years old with low bone density were given either low dose estrogen (0.3 milligrams/day) along with progesterone or a placebo pill (no hormones were given to the placebo group). Both groups were given supplemental vitamin D and enough supplemental calcium to bring their calcium intake to over 1,000 milligrams daily. After 3.5 years, bone density in the spine increased by 5.2 percent in women who adhered to the combined hormone and nutrient supplementation treatment. This increase was roughly equivalent to that seen in women on higher dose hormone replacement therapy. (Women in the placebo group maintained their bone density, but it did not increase.) Symptoms related to low dose hormone replacement therapy were mild and short lived. Based on their results, the researchers concluded that *low dose HRT* with estrogen and progesterone *combined with adequate calcium and vitamin D* offers bone-sparing effects similar or superior to that provided by higher dose HRT regimens.[3]

While estrogen replacement therapy does offer bone protection, compliance rates are poor. It's estimated that only 15 percent of North American women are on hormone replacement therapy. And only 40 percent of women who are prescribed estrogen actually fill out their prescriptions. Furthermore, studies have revealed that 20 percent of women stop taking estrogen within nine months. Concerns about breast cancer risk, discomfort from PMS-like symptoms, or the sheer fact that taking hormone replacement can be a complicated procedure are a few reasons why women choose not to take estrogen or discontinue treatment.[4] For women who choose not to take estrogen, other drug-based options for osteoporosis prevention and treatment are discussed below.

BIPHOSPHONATES

This new class of non-hormonal drugs offers post-menopausal women with low bone density or osteoporosis a useful alternative to HRT. Biphosphonate drugs prevent bone loss by binding to the bone surface and inhibiting the activity of the osteoclasts, the cells that strip down old bone. In a nutshell, these drugs work by preventing bone breakdown. It seems that biphosphonates can actually decrease the number and life-span of osteoclasts. The end result is that the balance between bone breakdown and formation tips in favour of bone formation.

Didrocal™ (etidronate and calcium carbonate)

This bisphosphonate-calcium combination treatment is taken in 90-day cycles. For the first 14 days a 400-milligram tablet of etidronate (the biphosphonate drug) is taken. Then a 500-milligram calcium carbonate pill is taken for 76 days. Etidronate interferes with the osteoclast cells to reduce bone breakdown, and the calcium provides the raw material the body uses to form bone. Studies have shown that cyclic treatment with etidronate and calcium increases bone density and decreases the risk of spine fractures.[5] Etidronate is given in an on-off cycle because it is known that daily, long-term use can cause structural abnormalities in bone. Common side effects associated with this drug regime include nausea and diarrhea. Post-menopausal women who are taking Didrocal™ must make sure they get at least 1,500 milligrams of calcium daily from their diet and supplements (including the calcium supplied by the Didrocal™ regime), as well as 400 international units (IU) of vitamin D.

Fosamax™ (aldendronate)

Chances are you've heard about this biphosphonate drug, or perhaps you're already taking it. Studies of women who are within five years of menopause show that 5 milligrams of Fosamax™ each day can maintain bone density in 85 percent of treated women. Fosamax™ and estrogen appear equivalent in their ability to preserve bone in the hip, spine, and throughout the body after two years of treatment.[6] In Canada, a daily Fosamax™ dose of five milligrams is an accepted treatment for the prevention of osteoporosis.

I have many clients taking Fosamax™ who are pleased with their bone density results. There are, however, a couple of disadvantages to taking Fosamax™. First of all, you must take the drug on an empty stomach, with a glass of water—so you generally have to take it first thing in the morning and then wait at least 30 minutes before eating breakfast. If you take Fosamax™ with food, coffee, or juice you won't absorb any of the medication. The second drawback is the fact that you have to stay upright after taking the pill (you can't go back to bed!). Staying upright prevents the pill from coming back from your stomach into your esophagus where it can cause severe irritation and possibly ulcers. However, in view of the positive benefits to bone health achieved with Fosamax™, most women consider these small sacrifices to make.

Selective Estrogen Receptor Modulators (SERMs)

Considerable effort has been applied to the development of what might be called "designer estrogens." These drugs offer all the beneficial effects of estrogen (bone protection, cholesterol lowering, hot flash reduction), without causing any of its negative effects (increased breast cancer risk, endometrial bleeding). The first of these drugs to be developed was Tamoxifen, which has been used for many years to help prevent the recurrence of breast cancer in women. While Tamoxifen acts as an anti-estrogen in the breast, it acts like an estrogen in bone and does increase bone density in postmenopausal women (but to a lesser extent than regular estrogen and Fosamax™.) However, it also acts like an estrogen in the uterus and stimulates the growth of endometrial tissue, which may increase the risk of endometrial cancer. For this reason

Tamoxifen is not used to prevent osteoporosis. It may, however, offer women with breast cancer some bone protection.

Newer SERMs such as raloxifene and droloxifene act as anti-estrogens in the breast and the uterus. That means they don't stimulate the growth of breast or uterine cells. And they do appear to offer some of the favourable effects of estrogen on bone and blood cholesterol levels. Unlike estrogen, however, they don't relieve hot flashes or vaginal dryness. Clinical studies in post-menopausal women indicate that a daily raloxifene dose of 60 milligrams prevents bone loss without stimulating endometrial tissue.[7] Raloxifene is available as Evista® in Canada.

Ideally, every woman's goal should be to slow down, as much as possible, age related bone loss during her thirties, forties, and fifties so that bone-sparing medication is not necessary after menopause. Unfortunately, some women, either because of medical problems, lack of knowledge, or difficult life circumstances, are not able to take effective action during the pre-menopausal years and do develop low bone density. These women do require drugs to halt bone loss and reduce the risk of bone fracture. Yet, even if you are taking medication now, diet and nutritional supplements can still influence your bone density. If you read my "Research File" on page 107 you learned that adding calcium supplements to low dose estrogen therapy is equally effective at preserving bone as high dose hormone regimens. Here's a look at the nutritional strategies that can help slow down bone loss before and after menopause. Start paying attention now! It's never too late.

dietary approaches

SOY FOODS

Once again the humble soybean makes an appearance. By now you might be wondering if there's anything that soybeans can't do. I must admit, I'm hard pressed to come up with an answer (wait until you read about their cholesterol lowering ability in Chapter 9). If you've read Chapter 1, on hot flashes, you've already learned a lot about the medicinal properties of soy foods. Soybeans contain naturally occurring compounds called isoflavones, a type of plant estrogen. Genistein and daidzein are the most active isoflavones in soy and have been the focus of much research. Isoflavones have a chemical structure similar to that of estrogen and because of this they are able to bind to estrogen receptors in the body. In fact, genistein has a very strong affinity for certain estrogen receptors called beta-receptors. It is the action of isoflavones on estrogen receptors in the bone that scientists believe may be responsible for soy's potential bone preserving effect.

The interest in soybeans and osteoporosis began when researchers observed that populations who consume soy foods on a regular basis report much lower rates of hip fracture. Since then, soy foods and their naturally occurring phytoestrogens have been the focus of many studies. While some studies find that soy consumption has no effect on bone loss, others show soy to have a significant bone saving effect.

In November 1999 I attended the Third International Symposium on Soy Foods and Health in Washington D.C. Top researchers in the soy field presented their findings regarding the effect of soy on bones. The news looks promising! A three-month study conducted at Iowa State University found that 40 grams of phytoestrogen-rich soy protein powder prevented bone loss in post-menopausal women. On the other hand, women in this study who were given whey protein powder (a protein made from milk) instead of the soy showed significant bone loss in the lower spine.

Another study from Dr. Ken Setchell's group at the Department of Obstetrics and Gynecology, Internal Medicine and Pediatrics at the University of Cinncinati's College of Medicine found that 60 to 70 milligrams of soy isoflavones consumed daily in the form of So Good™ soy beverage and soy nuts significantly decreased bone turnover in post-menopausal women. The researchers found that in these women osteoblast activity (bone building) increased by 10.2 percent and osteoclast activity (bone breakdown) activity decreased by 13.9 percent. Reduced bone loss was seen after only four weeks of eating soy foods.[8]

The studies that have found a bone sparing effect give participants enough soy foods to supply 70 to 90 milligrams of isoflavones daily. And it is also important to note that in these studies isoflavones are consumed in two doses (in other words, twice daily). Depending on what kind of soy food you eat, your blood level of genistein will peak anywhere from four to eight hours later. If you want to keep your blood genistein levels high, it makes sense to eat soy foods in the morning and once again in the afternoon or evening. Soy foods vary with respect to the amount of isoflavones they contain. Even the same type of food made by different manufacturers can differ in isoflavone content. You'll find a general guide to soy foods and their isoflavone content on page 7.

PROTEIN FOODS

Eating too much protein may be part of the reason why North American women have high rates of osteoporosis, despite our moderate-to-high calcium intakes. Studies have shown that high levels of dietary protein cause calcium to be excreted by the kidneys. The effect of eating large quantities of protein is rapid, and it appears that the body doesn't correct for it by absorbing more calcium from food. People who consume very little calcium or who absorb very little calcium because of intestinal problems may find it especially important to take the protein effect into account.

It's estimated that the average North American overshoots the recommended daily intake for protein by more than 50 percent. And that doesn't take into account all those people following faddish high protein weight loss diets! I hate to think how those diets impact on calcium loss and bone health. But while eating very large amounts of protein may not be good for your bones, eating too little isn't healthy either. Protein is an important structural component of bone and studies have shown that eating too little might actually increase the risk of hip fracture. The Iowa Women's Health Study found that dietary protein protected post-menopausal women from hip fracture. And it appeared that animal protein, rather than vegetable protein, accounted for this protection. Women who ate the most protein, while staying within the recommended daily intake levels, had a 69 percent reduced risk of hip fracture compared to women who ate the least.

Extra protein may also help women with hip fractures. A Swiss study of 82 patients with recent hip fracture showed that a 20 gram protein supplement taken daily reduced bone loss and shortened hospital stay. In addition, the study participants experienced lower complication and death rates immediately after surgery and for six months afterwards. This effect is not seen in hip fracture patients who are not given extra protein.[9]

Although the protein issue is controversial, it does seem clear that it's important to be getting enough. Women at risk for protein deficiency include:
- Those who live alone and don't often cook meat, chicken, or fish.
- Those who frequently grab a quick meal during the day—a bagel, pasta, a low fat frozen dinner.

- Vegetarians who do not regularly incorporate high quality vegetable protein sources into their diet.
- Those who engage in heavy exercise and fall into any of the above categories.

How much protein do you need? Here's a look at the Recommended Daily Allowances (RDAs) for protein for adult females.

PROTEIN RDAS FOR ADULT FEMALES
(GRAMS PER KILOGRAM OF BODY WEIGHT)

No regular exercise	0.8
Regular exercise	1.2
Heavy exercise	1.2–1.7

To calculate your actual protein requirements for the day, you need to multiply your weight (in kilograms) by your RDA for protein. To start, obtain your weight in kilograms by multiplying your weight in pounds by 0.45. For example, a 135 pound woman weighs 61 kilograms (135 x 0.45 = 61). Now let's say that this woman does not exercise. Her RDA for protein is therefore 0.8 grams per kilogram of body weight. That means she needs 49 grams of protein each day (61 x 0.8 grams). If this same woman was exercising three or four times per week, she would need to eat 73 grams of protein daily (61 x 1.2 grams). If you're wondering how much food you have to eat to get this much protein, here's a look.

PROTEIN CONTENT OF COMMON FOODS (GRAMS)

Meat, 3 ounces (90 grams)	21–25
Poultry, 3 ounces (90 grams)	21
Salmon, 3 ounces (90 grams)	25
Sole, 3 ounces (90 grams)	17
Tuna, canned and drained, 1/2 cup (125 ml)	30
Egg, 1 whole	6
Legumes, 1/2 cup (125 ml)	8
Milk, 1 cup (250 ml)	8
Yogurt, 3/4 cup (175 ml)	8
Cheese, cheddar, 1 ounce (30 g)	10

Vegetables, 1/2 cup (125 ml)	2
Bread, 1 slice	2
Rice, pasta, cooked, 1/2 cup (125 ml)	2

ALCOHOL

Here's another dietary factor that can have both a positive and negative effect on bone health. Many studies have determined that chronic alcohol abuse causes low bone density. Alcohol acts directly on your bones and suppresses bone formation. Consuming alcohol also increases the risk of falls in post-menopausal women and is associated with an increased incidence of hip fractures.

But there is also evidence to suggest that moderate alcohol drinking (one or two drinks a day) may actually increase bone density. Many population studies have found that a moderate pattern of drinking is linked with higher bone densities. It does seem odd that alcohol might actually stimulate bone building. It turns out that alcohol increases estrogen levels in the blood, and estrogen, as you know, has a bone sparing action. The famous Nurses' Health Study conducted by Harvard University researchers investigated alcohol use and bone health in 188 post-menopausal women. They found that women who consumed 75 grams of alcohol each day had significantly higher bone density in the lower spine than non-drinkers. The study showed that as alcohol intake rose from none to 75 grams, bone density increased in proportion. This suggests that women may also benefit from taking less than 75 grams of alcohol daily.[10]

NUTRITION TIP

How much alcohol does it contain?

If you want to know how to keep your alcohol intake below 75 grams daily, it helps to know just how much of it is present in everyday drinks.

ALCOHOL CONTENT OF COMMON BEVERAGES (GRAMS)

Beer, regular, 12 oz. (375 ml) bottle	14–16
Beer, light, 12 oz. (375 ml) bottle	11
Wine, red or white, 6 oz. (187 ml)	16
Liquor, 80 proof, 1.5 oz. (45 ml)	14

When you consider the fact that a moderate intake of alcohol (one or two drinks daily) increases the risk of breast cancer (read Chapter 10 for more on this topic), I certainly don't recommend that non-drinkers start drinking. There are plenty of other bone building factors that you can incorporate into your life (like calcium, vitamin D, and exercise, for starters). But if you do enjoy a drink or two each day, you'll be pleased to know that it might help preserve your bone density.

CAFFEINE

Drinking coffee, tea, or cola increases the amount of calcium your kidneys excrete in the urine. Increased calcium excretion continues up to three hours after consuming caffeine. It's been estimated that every six-ounce cup (175 millilitres) of coffee leaches 48 milligrams of calcium from your body.

One study found a significant relationship between increasing caffeine intakes and lower bone density in 980 post-menopausal women. The effects of caffeine are likely most detrimental for women who are not meeting their calcium requirements. Another study from Tufts University in Boston found that women who consumed less than 800 milligrams of calcium and 450 milligrams of caffeine (about three small cups of coffee) daily had significantly lower bone densities than women who consumed the same amount of caffeine but more than 800 milligrams of calcium.[11] Coffee drinking has also been associated with a greater risk of hip fracture in older women.

The bottom line on caffeine is quite simple:

- If you drink coffee make sure you're meeting your calcium requirement of 1,000 to 1,500 milligrams daily.
- Don't consume more than 450 milligrams of caffeine a day.
- Add three tablespoons (45 millilitres) of milk (this amount contains 58 milligrams of calcium) or calcium fortified soy beverage to every cup of coffee you drink.

Here are a few tips to help you decaffeinate your day:

- Eliminate caffeine containing beverages after noon (that means you can keep your morning wake up cup!). Instead try water, herbal tea, vegetable juice, milk, or a glass of soy beverage.
- Replace coffee with tea, which has substantially less caffeine.
- Instead of plain coffee, try a calcium-rich latte made with milk or fortified soy beverage.

SODIUM

Like caffeine, sodium also causes your kidneys to excrete calcium. For every 500-milligram increase in your sodium intake, you must eat an additional 40 milligrams of calcium to make up for the increased loss. A study in post-menopausal women determined that a maximum daily intake of 2,000 milligrams of sodium and 1,000 milligrams of caffeine minimized bone loss.[12] (By the way, 2,000 milligrams of sodium is the amount that's found in about 3/4 teaspoons (3 millilitres) of salt.)

Although we do need some salt every day, we need very little. Salt is made of sodium and chloride, both of which are needed to help maintain water balance in our body. We continually lose sodium through sweat and urine. The more active we are or the warmer the weather, the more sodium we must replace from the diet. But here's the kicker—it only takes about 115 milligrams (or 1/20 of a teaspoon) of salt to meet the daily needs of sedentary people living in temperate climates. The average Canadian consumes about 1 and 3/4 teaspoons (4025 milligrams) of salt each day, almost 40 times more than we need!

To help yourself cut back on sodium I recommend that you avoid the salt shaker at the table, minimize the use of salt in cooking, and try to buy commercial food products that are low in added salt. Eating fewer processed foods is one of the best things you can do to cut back on sodium. That's because most of the salt we eat every day comes from processed and prepared foods. It might surprise you to learn that for most of us, only one-quarter of our daily sodium intake comes from the salt shaker.

Here's how much salt is found in commercial foods (remember, you're aiming to consume less than one teaspoon—5 millilitres—daily).

ADDED SALT CONTENT OF COMMON COMMERCIAL FOODS (TEASPOONS)
Soups

Chicken noodle soup, 1 cup (250 ml)	1/2
Cup of Noodles	3/4
Low sodium soups	1/20

Crackers

Soda crackers, 8	1/4

Processed meats

Bologna, 2 slices	2/3
Ham, 3 ounces (90 g)	1/2
Wiener, 1	1/4

Snack foods

Pretzels, 1 cup (250 ml)	1/3
Popcorn, salted, 3 cups (750 ml)	1/4

Canned foods

Peas, canned, 1/2 cup (125 ml)	1/8
Pasta sauce, 1/2 cup (125 ml)	1/2
Pork and beans, canned, 1 cup (250 ml)	1/2

Packaged foods

Peas, frozen in sauce, 1/2 cup (125 ml)	1/4
Rice & Sauce, 1 cup (250 ml)	1/2
Pasta & Sauce, 1 cup (250 ml)	1/2

Fast food

Burger (Big Mac)	1/2
1 piece Crispy KFC, breast	1/2
French fries, large order	1/4

vitamins and minerals

CALCIUM

The fact that calcium is the most abundant mineral in the body and that 99 percent of it is housed within the bones and teeth underlines the importance of dietary calcium to bone health. During the bone building process, the osteoblast cells secrete bone mineral (consisting of calcium and phosphorus) which strengthens the bone. This mineral matures into hyroxyapatite, a compound responsible for the strength and rigidity of bones. By making it possible for the osteoblasts to provide structural integrity to bones, dietary calcium plays a critical role in preventing osteoporosis.

Think back to what happens to your bones if your diet is low in calcium. One percent of your body's calcium circulates in your bloodstream and is vital to your heart, nervous system, and muscles. Your body keeps this circulating pool of calcium at a constant level. If your diet is lacking calcium and your blood calcium level drops, you'll recall that your parathyroid gland releases parathyroid hormone (PTH). This hormone then goes to work to return calcium to your blood. It makes your kidneys stop excreting calcium and it works with vitamin D to release calcium from your bones into your blood. So when you shortchange your diet, you shortchange your bones too.

How much calcium do you need?

In August 1997, the Food and Nutrition Board of the National Academy of Sciences, a panel of experts from the United States and Canada, released new recommended intakes for calcium (also for vitamin D, magnesium, and phosphorus). The need to revise the recommended daily intake for calcium became evident after years of research revealed how much calcium is needed for optimal bone health. The old recommendations were based on how much calcium was needed to prevent a deficiency. We now know how much of the mineral is required to prevent osteoporosis and bone fracture. Here's a look at how much you and your family members need:

RECOMMENDED CALCIUM INTAKES (MILLIGRAMS)

Children, 4 to 8	800
Children, 9 to 12	1,300
Teenagers, 13 to 18	1,300
Adults, 19 to 50	1,000
Adults, over 50	1,200–1,500
Pregnant women	1,000

Getting more calcium into your diet

Ideally, I encourage clients to get as much calcium as possible from food. Unlike calcium pills, many calcium-rich foods provide other important bone building nutrients like vitamin D, magnesium, and potassium. One study found that spinal bone loss was significantly lower in premenopausal women who used milk products to raise their calcium intake from 900 milligrams to 1,500 milligrams.[13] If you suspect you may not be getting as much calcium as you need, see my list of calcium-rich foods below to help you boost your intake.

CALCIUM CONTENT OF CALCIUM-RICH FOODS (MILLIGRAMS)
Dairy foods

Milk (Lactaid or plain milk), 1 cup (250 ml)	300
Milk (Neilson TruTaste), 1 cup (250 ml)	360
Milk (Neilson TruCalcium), 1 cup (250 ml)	420
Carnation Instant Breakfast, with 1 cup (250 ml) milk	540
Chocolate milk, 1 cup (250 ml)	285
Cheese, cheddar, 1.5 oz (45 g)	300
Cheese, Swiss or gruyère, 1.5 oz. (45 g)	480
Cheese, mozzarella, 1.75 oz (50 g)	269
Cheese, cottage, 1/2 cup (125 ml)	75
Cheese, ricotta, 1/2 cup (125 ml)	255
Evaporated milk, 1/2 cup (125 ml)	350
Light sour cream, 1/4 cup (50 ml)	120
Pudding, low fat Healthy Choice, 1/2 cup (125 ml)	110
Skim milk powder, dry, 3 tbsp. (45 ml)	155
Yogurt, plain, 3/4 cup (175 ml)	300
Yogurt, fruit, 3/4 cup (175 ml)	250

Legumes

Soybeans, cooked, 1 cup (250 ml)	175
Soybeans, roasted, 1/4 cup (50 ml)	60
Soy beverage, 1 cup (250 ml)	100

Soy beverage, fortified, 1 cup (250 ml)	300 to 330
Baked beans, 1 cup (250 ml)	150
Black beans, cooked, 1 cup (250 ml)	102
Kidney beans, cooked, 1 cup (250 ml)	69
Lentils, cooked, 1 cup (250 ml)	37
Tempeh, cooked, 1 cup (250 ml)	154
Tofu, raw firm, with calcium sulphate, 4 oz. (120 g)	260
Tofu, raw, regular, with calcium sulphate, 4 oz. (120 g)	130

Fish

Sardines, 8 small (with bones)	165
Salmon, 1/2 can drained (with bones)	225

Vegetables

Broccoli, raw, 1 cup (250 ml)	42
Broccoli, cooked, 1 cup (250 ml)	94
Bok choy, cooked, 1 cup (250 ml)	158
Collard greens, cooked, 1 cup (250 ml)	357
Kale, cooked, 1 cup (250 ml)	179
Rutabaga, cooked, 1/2 cup (125 ml)	57
Swiss chard, raw, 1 cup (250 ml)	21
Swiss chard, cooked, 1 cup (250 ml)	102
Okra, cooked, 1 cup (250 ml)	176

Fruits

Currants, 1/2 cup (125 ml)	60
Figs, 5 medium	135
Orange, 1 medium	50

Nuts

Almonds, 1/4 cup (50 ml)	100
Brazil nuts, 1/4 cup (50 ml)	65
Hazelnuts, 1/4 cup (50 ml)	65

Molasses

Blackstrap molasses, 2 tbsp. (25 ml)	288
Fancy molasses, 2 tbsp. (25 ml)	70

FORTIFIED ORANGE JUICE

Oasis Florida Premium Orange Juice, 1 cup (250 ml)	300
Oasis Health Break (juice & milk cocktail), 1 cup (250 ml)	300
Tropicana Calcium Fortified Orange Juice, 1 cup (250 ml)	300
Minute Maid Calcium Fortified Orange Juice, 1 cup (250 ml)	300

Here are more ways to boost your calcium intake:

- If you use dairy products, aim for three servings daily.
- Cook hot cereal, rice, and grains in low fat milk or a calcium fortified soy beverage.
- Add milk to cream soups, puddings, egg dishes.
- Add skim milk powder to casseroles, soups, shakes, meat loaf, French toast, muffin batters, breads, mashed potatoes, and dips—1/4 cup (50 millilitres) packs in 210 milligrams of calcium!
- Use evaporated 2% or evaporated skim milk instead of regular milk in pudding, cream soups, and cream sauces—1 cup (250 millilitres) contains 700 milligrams of calcium.
- Top a baked potato with 1/4 cup (50 ml) low fat sour cream for an additional 70 milligrams of calcium.
- Try an instant breakfast drink made with 1 cup (250 millilitres) skim milk to gain 400 milligrams of calcium.
- Eat *at least* two servings of calcium-rich vegetables every day—one serving is 1/2 cup (125 millilitres) of cooked vegetables.

Boosting calcium absorption

On average we absorb about 30 percent of the calcium we consume in our diet. In other words, if you are getting 1,000 milligrams of calcium from food each day, your body is absorbing about 300 milligrams of that. But you needn't worry. The scientists who set the RDA for calcium took into account the fact that our bodies absorb calcium inefficiently. What you should worry about, however, are factors in your diet that make your body absorb calcium even less effectively. Here's a look at dietary factors that limit calcium absorption:

- Large amounts of phytates (a type of fibre). Phytates in wheat bran and other grains can bind with calcium and limit its absorption.
- Oxalic acid in spinach and some other vegetables. (You may have noticed in the chart of calcium containing foods above that cooking green vegetables boosts their calcium content. That's because cooking releases some calcium that's bound to oxalic acid.)
- Too much phosphorus in the diet.
- Taking iron with calcium-rich foods (iron competes with calcium for absorption).
- Drinking tea with a meal rich in calcium. Natural compounds in tea known as tannins inhibit calcium absorption.
- A lack of vitamin D (as you've read above, vitamin D stimulates the intestines to absorb dietary calcium).

Calcium absorption is also affected by our body's need for the mineral. During the rapid growth of childhood, the body absorbs about 75 percent of dietary calcium. During pregnancy, absorption may be as high as 60 percent. In general, the younger we are, the more calcium we absorb. After menopause, calcium absorption can be as low as 20 percent.

What about a supplement?

Studies do support the idea of using calcium supplements to minimize your odds of osteoporosis. Researchers at the University of Texas Southwestern Medical Center in Dallas found that a 400 milligram calcium citrate supplement taken twice daily increased bone density in healthy post-menopausal women. Women taking the calcium pills experienced no loss of bone density in the radial shaft (one of two bones in the forearm), neck, or lower spine after two years of treatment. In contrast, women in the placebo group experienced a 2.38 percent reduction in the bone density of the lower spine.

Other studies have found that calcium supplements can prevent bone loss in premenopausal women. Scientists at the University of Massachusetts studied 98 premenopausal women (average age, 39 years) for three years. Those who received 500 milligrams of calcium carbonate increased their bone density by 0.3 percent per year. The women in the placebo group lost bone at a rate of 0.4 percent per year in the hip and 0.7 percent per year in the neck. According to the researchers, if this rate of bone density loss occurred throughout the years between 30 and 50, the total loss would be between 8 and 14 percent—a loss that translates into a doubled or tripled risk of hip fracture. A number of studies have also shown that older women (and men) who take calcium and vitamin D supplements have a lower incidence of nonvertebral fractures.[14]

By now you're probably thinking you'd better visit your local pharmacy to pick up a calcium supplement. And chances are, you're probably right. Recent surveys have found that most Canadians get a mere 1.6 servings of milk products each day. That translates into 480 milligrams of calcium—a far cry from 1,000 or 1,200 milligrams. Sure, there's broccoli and almonds and tofu. But let's be truthful here. Do you really eat tofu on a daily basis? Are you willing to eat five cups of cooked broccoli to make up for your missing 500 milligrams of calcium? I do realize I'm being a little extreme to make my point, but the truth is, many women are not meeting their daily calcium needs and should be taking a calcium supplement. It can be especially difficult to meet your calcium goals if you're lactose intolerant (you can't digest a sugar found in milk, called lactose), following a vegetarian diet, or if you have poor eating habits. I find that in many situations, I recommend calcium supplements to my clients, as they represent the only way that I can ensure a woman will meet her calcium needs.

To help you determine your need for a calcium supplement, use my "300 Milligram Rule." One milk serving gives you about 300 milligrams of calcium. That means that in order to get 1,200 milligrams of calcium, you need to eat four milk servings. For every serving you don't get and don't replace with other calcium-rich foods, you need to take 300 milligrams of elemental calcium in supplemental form. But before you rush off to the health food store, keep in mind that there are a few things to look for when buying a supplement.

Choosing a quality supplement

If you've been to the pharmacy or health food store and found yourself overwhelmed by all the different types of calcium supplements, you're not alone. Many of my clients have described their frustration about calcium supplements. Should you choose calcium carbonate or calcium citrate? Is a 600-milligram pill better than two 300-milligram tablets? What about added vitamin D and magnesium? I'm sure that many of you know what I mean. To help make your next calcium shopping experience stress-free, follow these guidelines for choosing a high quality supplement.

Look at the source There are many types of calcium supplements on the shelf. These are the most common types:

- **Calcium carbonate** Only about 10 to 30 percent of this form of calcium is absorbed. The amount you absorb depends on how much stomach acid you have. As you age, your stomach produces less hydrochloric acid. Always take calcium carbonate supplements with meals to increase their absorption. Do not take calcium carbonate at bedtime, unless you take it with a night-time snack. Calcium carbonate is not the best choice for older adults or people on medications that block acid production. On the plus side, calcium carbonate is the most inexpensive type of calcium.

NUTRITION TIP

Testing your calcium carbonate pill

Since a calcium carbonate supplement needs to break down completely before it can be absorbed, I recommend that you test your brand to determine how quickly it disintegrates.

- Drop your calcium carbonate tablet into a glass of vinegar.
- If most of the tablet hasn't disintegrated within 30 minutes, you need to switch to another brand that will disintegrate that quickly.

If you're using a "chewable" calcium supplement, disintegration is not a big concern, since the act of chewing helps to break the pill down.

- **Calcium citrate** You absorb about 30 percent of the calcium in a calcium citrate pill, so this form is more available to your bones than calcium carbonate. Calcium citrate is therefore a better choice for anyone over the age of 50. Calcium citrate malate is one of the most highly absorbable (and expensive) forms of calcium. Calcium citrate supplements are well absorbed with meals or on an empty stomach.

- **Calcium chelates (HVP chelates)** These are supplements that contain calcium that's bound to an amino acid (amino acids are the most basic forms of protein). In the case of HVP chelate, the amino acid is extracted from vegetable proteins. Some manufacturers claim that up to 75 percent of calcium in the chelate form is absorbed by the body.
- **Effervescent calcium supplements** These contain calcium carbonate and often other forms of more absorbable calcium. For this reason they may be better absorbed by some people. And because the calcium in these supplements starts disintegrating before it reaches the digestive tract, it may be absorbed more quickly. Dissolve effervescent calcium supplements in water or orange juice.
- **Bone meal (hydroxyapatite, dolomite, or oyster shell)** Taking a calcium supplement made from any of these sources is not recommended because some products have been found to contain trace quantities of contaminants such as lead and mercury.

Look at the elemental calcium   The list of ingredients will alert you to how much elemental calcium each pill will give you. The amount of elemental calcium is what you use to calculate your daily intake. The label may state that this is a 500-milligram supplement, but when you look at the ingredient list on the bottle, you may find the product contains only 350 milligrams of elemental calcium. This amount, and not the 500-milligram amount, will determine how many tablets you need to take to get your recommended calcium dose. For instance, if you need to supplement your diet with 1,000 milligrams of calcium daily, you would take three of these pills, not two.

Look for vitamin D and magnesium   Choose a calcium formula that includes vitamin D and magnesium. These nutrients work in tandem with calcium to promote optimal bone health. For instance, vitamin D increases calcium absorption in your intestines by as much as 30 to 80 percent.

How much calcium is too much?

The daily upper limit for calcium intake is 2,500 milligrams. In most healthy people, this amount will not cause any side effects. The major risks you run from getting too much calcium include kidney stones, constipation, and gas. To lower your risk of kidney stones, take your calcium supplements with a large glass of water. Drinking sufficient water with the supplement helps to prevent calcium buildup in the kidneys.

You might be interested to learn that people who take 1,300 milligrams of calcium daily in supplemental form, as compared to people who take 500 milligrams, have fewer kidney stones made from oxalate (oxalic acid). High amounts of calcium in the intestines can bind to oxalates in the diet (found in spinach, rhubarb, and other vegetables), preventing its absorption and reducing the amount that eventually reaches the kidneys to cause stones. But in people who have a history of kidney stones, excessive intakes of calcium can increase the risk of stone formation. At intakes higher than 2,500 milligrams, too much calcium can reach the kidneys for excretion in the urine.

Very high intakes of calcium from milk, fortified beverages, and supplements can cause a condition called milk-alkali syndrome. In this condition the level of calcium in the bloodstream becomes so high that calcium "leaches" into body tissues and destroys them. As long as you stay at or below the upper limit of 2,500 milligrams daily calcium intake, you don't have to worry about milk-alkali syndrome.

Lactose intolerance

If you suffer gastric distress after drinking a glass of milk, chances are you're not alone. In my private practice it's not uncommon for me to hear people complain of difficulty digesting lactose, the natural sugar found in dairy products. The fact that 70 percent of the world's population has difficulty digesting lactose has led some researchers to believe that lactose intolerance is normal and lactose tolerance is the abnormal condition. Lactose intolerance is caused by low levels of lactase, the enzyme in the small intestines that breaks down the milk sugar and makes it ready for absorption. If lactose remains undigested in the gut it draws water into the intestines, which can lead to diarrhea. Also, bacteria in the intestinal tract will begin to ferment the undigested lactose, causing bloating, gas, and discomfort.

Lactose intolerance is more common among people of Asian, African, and South American descent. Many individuals with these origins lose the ability to produce lactase when they're children. Difficulty digesting lactose can also occur when other gastrointestinal problems are present, such as celiac disease, irritable bowel syndrome, Crohn's Disease, or a gastrointestinal infection. In these cases, the intolerance is often temporary and disappears when bowel health returns to normal.

Just because you have a lactose intolerance doesn't mean you have to give up calcium-rich dairy products. Most people with a mild to moderate lactose intolerance can handle yogurt quite well and can tolerate milk in one-half cup (125-millilitre) servings.

The bacteria in yogurt actually digest some of the lactose so you end up with a food that has considerably less lactose than a glass of milk. For a list of dairy products that contain lower amounts of lactose, check the following Nutrition Tip.

NUTRITION TIP

Dairy products with less lactose

Avoiding lactose? Here's a ranking of foods according to their lactose content. If you have a strong lactose intolerance, also make sure to read ingredient lists on packaged and processed food labels. If you see milk, milk solids, cheese flavour, or whey curds in the list of ingredients, there's lactose present.

High lactose
- Condensed milk
- Evaporated milk
- Processed cheese

Moderate lactose
- Cottage cheese, 2%
- Feta cheese
- Fluid milk
- Goat's milk
- Ice cream
- Mozzarella cheese
- Ricotta cheese
- Swiss cheese
- Yogurt, low fat

Low lactose
- Brie cheese
- Butter
- Cheddar cheese
- Cottage cheese, 1%
- Cream cheese
- Lactaid milk

Lactose free (non-dairy products)
- Calcium fortified orange juice
- Calcium fortified rice based beverages
- Calcium fortified soy beverages

Some people, however, have severe lactose intolerance and must avoid all sources of lactose. While a diet without dairy products can still offer plenty of calcium, vitamin D, which is so important for adequate calcium absorption, is often more of a problem. Calcium fortified orange juice, tofu, broccoli, leafy greens, almonds, and legumes are all good sources of calcium but none of them have vitamin D. Continue reading to find out how to get enough vitamin D.

VITAMIN D

By now you've heard and read from many sources besides just this book that too little dietary calcium makes bones brittle and increases the risk for osteoporosis. But experts also blame a silent epidemic of vitamin D deficiency. The main reason for this nutrient deficiency is the fact that most foods have little or no natural vitamin D and only a few foods are actually fortified with the vitamin.

Vitamin D acts like a hormone in your body (remember from Chapter 1 that a hormone is any compound manufactured in one part of the body that affects another part). The active form of vitamin D is made in your liver but acts on your intestines, your kidneys, and your bone. As I mentioned earlier, vitamin D raises blood levels of calcium in three ways—it stimulates your intestines to absorb more dietary calcium, it tells your kidneys to retain calcium, and it withdraws calcium from your bones. Vitamin D works alone in the intestinal tract and in the kidneys and bones, in tandem with parathyroid hormone. The end result of vitamin D activity is that more calcium and phosphorus become available for bone growth—these minerals are supplied to the bones via the blood, and are deposited as new bone hardens, or mineralizes.

As you can see, vitamin D's main job is to maintain your blood calcium in the normal range. If you're not eating enough calcium-rich foods, then vitamin D removes calcium from your bones to keep your blood level constant. Simply put, if you're lacking vitamin D you are not absorbing enough calcium to meet your needs, regardless of how much calcium you consume. A vitamin D deficiency will speed up bone loss and increase the risk of fracture at a younger age.

Vitamin D is different from any other essential nutrient in that our bodies can synthesize it with the help of sunlight. When ultraviolet light from the sun reaches your skin, it becomes possible for your body, through a special chemical reaction, to convert a vitamin D precursor that's made from cholesterol into previtamin D3. This compound then makes its way to your liver where it's transformed into the active form of vitamin D (25-hydroxy vitamin D3). As you can see in the diagram, vitamin D in food must also be converted to an active form by the liver before it can go to work.

VITAMIN D SOURCES AND ACTIVATION

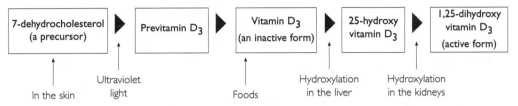

While exposing your skin to sunlight can provide most, or all, of the vitamin D your body needs, very little vitamin D synthesis occurs in the skin of many Canadians for months at a time because of our long winters. The situation is exacerbated by the fact that most of us work indoors. Researchers from Tufts University in Boston have demonstrated that blood levels of vitamin D do indeed fluctuate throughout the year. They are at their lowest point in February-March and at their highest in June-July.[15] But even in the summer, you might not be making enough vitamin D. Did you know that the sunscreen that protects you from skin cancer actually blocks the production of vitamin D? It's true. Suntan lotion with a sun protection factor (SPF) as low as 8 prevents 95 percent of your skin's vitamin D production. When it is sunny, you should expose your hands, face, and arms for 10 to 15 minutes, two or three times a week, without sunscreen, to help you meet your vitamin D needs. You can also now see how important it is to get plenty of vitamin D from food, not only in the winter but also in the summer months.

How much vitamin D do you need?

At the same time that it presented new recommendations for calcium intake (August 1997), the National Academy of Science released new intake guidelines for vitamin D. Based on current scientific understanding of vitamin D and bone health, recommended intakes for the vitamin were doubled for every age group. Here's how much you should be striving to get every day:

RECOMMENDED VITAMIN D INTAKES (INTERNATIONAL UNITS/IU)

0–50 years	200
51–70 years	400
71+ years	600

As you can see, the need to obtain vitamin D from food increases with age—older people make less vitamin D from sunlight. By the time the average person reaches the age of 70, the vitamin D precursor levels in the skin are three to four times lower than in a younger person.

Available evidence shows that post-menopausal women should consume 400 to 800 IU of vitamin D each day to minimize bone loss. Unfortunately, good food sources of vitamin D are few and far between. Vitamin D occurs naturally in egg yolks, liver, butter, and oily fish. Foods fortified with the vitamin include fluid milk, margarine, and some brands of soy and rice beverages. Take at look at how these foods impact your vitamin D intake:

VITAMIN D CONTENT OF FOODS (IU)

Herring, 3.5 ounces (100 g)	900
Salmon, canned, 3.5 ounces (100 g)	500
Sardines, 3.5 ounces (100 g)	300
Milk, fluid, 1 cup (250 ml)	100
Fortified soy beverage, 1 cup (250 ml)	100
Fortified rice beverage, 1 cup (250 ml)	100
Egg, 1 whole	24
Margarine, 1 tsp. (5 ml)	15

What about vitamin D supplements?

If you're over 50, if you don't drink at least two glasses of a fortified beverage every day, or if winter means little exposure to sunshine, then you should reach for a good quality multi-vitamin/mineral supplement to supply your D. The daily upper limit for vitamin D is 2,000 IU. Most supplements give you 400 IU. If you take calcium supplements, buy a product with vitamin D added. Fish oil is another way to get your vitamin D: one teaspoon (five millilitres) of cod liver oil packs 1,100 IU. If you take fish oil capsules, make sure you follow the manufacturer's dosage recommendations or better yet, get advice from a qualified dietitian or nutritionist. In addition to vitamin D, fish oil contains vitamin A. Both vitamins are fat soluble and are stored in your body. When taken in large doses over a period of time, fish oil supplements can cause vitamin A and vitamin D toxicity. Too much vitamin A can cause blurred vision, appetite loss, diarrhea, and skin rashes, and excess vitamin D can lead to kidney stones. So before you rush out to the health food store, consult your health care practitioner.

OTHER BONE BUILDING VITAMINS AND MINERALS

There's no doubt that calcium and vitamin D both play a crucial role in bone health. Without adequate calcium your bones cannot make an effective mineral complex (hydroxyapatite) that lends strength and rigidity to bones. And without enough vitamin D, your body cannot absorb the calcium it needs. But the story doesn't end here. Other nutrients are important for bone building as well. Together with calcium and vitamin D, they comprise the nutrient team that your body needs to orchestrate the continual process of bone remodeling.

Vitamin A

One of this vitamin's important jobs is to support growth and development, especially bone development. I told you earlier that in order to build new bone, the osteoclast cells must first undo parts of old bone. In order to accomplish this task, osteoclasts contain a sac of degradative enzymes. With the help of vitamin A, these enzymes break down old bone. The fact that bone growth relies on vitamin A is witnessed by the fact that children who are deficient in vitamin A fail to grow properly.

Vitamin A is found preformed in animal foods such as fortified milk, cheese, butter, eggs, and liver. But we also meet our vitamin A needs by eating bright orange and green fruits and vegetables. The beta-carotene in these plant foods is converted to vitamin A in the body. The best sources of beta-carotene include carrots (surprise, surprise), winter squash, sweet potatoes, spinach, broccoli, rapini, Romaine lettuce, apricots, peaches, mango, papaya, and cantaloupe.

Vitamin K

You've probably heard very little about this fat soluble vitamin. One of the reasons for its low profile is that a vitamin K deficiency is hardly ever seen. That's because the billions of bacteria in our intestinal tract synthesize this vitamin. Once we absorb this bacteria-manufactured vitamin K, it is stored in the liver. The vitamin is not a part of the bone mineral complex. Instead, your body needs it to make a bone protein called osteocalcin. Doctors can measure the amount of osteocalcin in your blood. A high level indicates that your osteoblasts are busy making new bone. Without enough vitamin K, the bones produce an abnormal protein that cannot bind to the minerals that give the bones their strength and defined form. The best food sources of vitamin K are leafy green vegetables, cabbage, milk, and liver.

When it comes to bone health, the importance of vitamin K should not be underestimated. The famous Nurses' Health Study from Harvard University found that women with the highest intake of vitamin K had a significantly lower rate of hip fracture as compared to women who consumed the least. And guess what? Eating lettuce was also linked with fewer hip fractures, because lettuce accounted for most of the vitamin K in the diet of the women with stronger bones. Those women who ate one or more servings of the leafy green each day (versus one or fewer servings a week) had a 45 percent lower risk of hip fracture.[16]

Phosphorus

This mineral is an important component of the bone mineral complex. In fact, about 85 percent of the phosphorus in the body is found in the bone. It appears that both too little dietary phosphorus and too much can result in bone loss. A high level in the blood causes the release of parathyroid hormone (PTH). And if you recall, PTH instructs your osteoclasts to release calcium into your bloodstream. Scientists believe that a longstanding imbalance of phosphorus and calcium, caused by too much dietary phosphorus and too little dietary calcium, may contribute to bone breakdown.

On the other hand, if your diet lacks phosphorus and your blood levels become low, your body will release the mineral from your bones in an effort to keep your blood level constant (the same way that calcium blood levels remain stable at the expense of your bone). One of the symptoms of a phosphorus deficiency is bone pain. A low blood phosphorus level can result from poor eating habits, intestinal malabsorption, and excessive use of antacids that bind to phosphorus, such as Maalox®, Diovol, Gelusil®, or Amphogel.

The daily recommended intake for phosphorus is 700 milligrams. Most of the phosphorus in our diet comes from additives in cheese, bakery products, processed meats, and soft drinks. Other food sources include wheat bran, milk, fish, eggs, poultry, beef, and pork. As you can probably guess, most people don't have a problem getting enough phosphorus. Perhaps vegans who use no commercial bread or other commercial products are at risk of a phosphorus deficiency. Everyone else, just make sure you meet your calcium requirements so that you keep these two minerals in balance.

Magnesium

One-half of the body's magnesium stores are in the bone. But before I continue, I'd like to clear up one piece of misinformation. Magnesium does not help your body absorb calcium! I can't begin to count the number of times I have heard this said. On occasion, I've even seen it written in books. Without magnesium, you'll absorb calcium just fine, but you won't form healthy bones. Your body needs magnesium to make parathyroid hormone, an important regulator of bone building. Animal studies show that a lack of dietary magnesium causes increased bone breakdown and decreased bone synthesis.

It's difficult to say to what extent magnesium plays a role in the development of osteoporosis since very few studies have actually looked at the effect of dietary magnesium intake on bone loss. Most of the studies that support the use of magnesium supplements have found that osteoporosis is more common in people who have other health problems that cause a magnesium deficiency, like alcoholism or hyperthyroidism. Interestingly, scientists have found that magnesium levels in bone are actually higher than normal, not lower, in people with osteoporosis.

Nonetheless, magnesium is an important nutrient for bone health and is also required for the smooth functioning of many other processes in the body. The recommended daily intake for women is 320 milligrams. The best food sources are wheat bran, whole grain breads, cereals and pasta, legumes, nuts, seeds, and leafy green vegetables. There's no question in my mind that most people need to step up their magnesium intake. If you stop eating refined starches like white bread and white pasta, and switch to whole grain products, you'll be making a good start. The fact that so many of my clients are lacking magnesium in their diet is why I recommend buying a calcium supplement that also includes magnesium. But too much supplemental magnesium can cause diarrhea. For this reason, I suggest you buy a calcium/magnesium supplement that offers these two nutrients in a two to one (2:1) ratio (two parts calcium to one part magnesium).

Boron

While there's no daily recommended intake for boron, studies suggest that higher intakes of this trace mineral may slow down loss of calcium, magnesium, and phosphorus from the urine. And that's not all. Boosting your boron intake may also increase your blood estrogen level. Scientists aren't exactly sure how boron keeps calcium in balance, but they think that boron is needed for activation of vitamin D.

A daily intake of 1.5 to 3 milligrams is probably more than adequate to meet your requirements for bone growth and development. Fruits and vegetables are the main food sources of boron, but their boron content will depend on how much of the mineral is in the soil they were grown in. If you want to take a supplement, 3 to 9 milligrams per day is a very safe amount. Intakes greater than 500 milligrams a day can cause nausea, vomiting, and diarrhea. Your best bet is to strive for at least five servings of fruits and vegetables each day.

Manganese, zinc, and copper

Your body uses these minerals to synthesize enzymes that are essential in making bone tissue. The impact of these nutrients on bone loss has been studied in post-menopausal women. In one two-year study, women who received a daily supplement of calcium, manganese, copper, and zinc had not experienced any bone loss of the spine by the end of the study. The placebo group, on the other hand, lost 3.5 percent of their bone mass.[17] Manganese is widely available in foods and deficiencies have not been seen in humans—you may want to check however, that your diet is supplying 5 milligrams daily, the amount used in this study (see Appendix 4, "A Quick Reference Guide to Vitamins and Minerals" to assess your manganese intake). Meat and tap water are your best bets for copper. When it comes to zinc, reach for wheat bran, wheat germ, oysters, seafood, lean red meat, and milk.

other lifestyle factors

THE IMPORTANCE OF EXERCISE

Regular exercise before the age of 30 helps women get a head start on building peak bone mass. In fact, studies have found that children who spend the most amount of time being physically active have stronger bones than those who are sedentary. But the effect of exercise doesn't stop once you've achieved your peak mass. Bone cells are constantly active, tearing up old bone and laying down new bone. Participating in weight bearing activities stimulates bones to increase in strength and density during the pre- and post-menopausal years. Weight bearing exercise is any exercise that forces you to support your own body weight and/or additional weight (as in weight training). Swimming and cycling are not considered weight bearing exercise since in the case of swimming, your weight is supported by the water, and in the case of cycling, by the bike! Brisk walking, jogging, stair climbing, and strength training are all good examples of weight bearing activities. One study found that post-menopausal women who worked out three times a week for nine months actually increased their bone mass by 5.2 percent.

If your exercise routine includes weight training, that's fabulous—and if it doesn't, you should consider adding this form of exercise to your routine. Researchers have learned that weight training also has a protective effect on bone density in women. Compared to women who didn't exercise, women who worked out with weights for one hour three times a week gained bone mass, to the tune of 1.6 percent. The non-exercisers actually lost 3.6 percent of the bone mass in their spine over the course of the study.[18]

If you have osteoporosis, a safe exercise program can help you slow bone loss, improve posture and balance, and build muscle strength and tone. The benefits of exercise can reduce your risk of falling and fracturing a bone.

Your best bet is to incorporate a mix of activities into your week. Aim to enjoy four sessions of weight bearing activities each week, and two or three workouts with weights. If you have never used weights before, be sure to consult a certified personal trainer. Personal trainers work in fitness clubs and many will come to your home. They'll design a safe and effective program for you. And don't worry, you won't need a basement full of exercise equipment. Some of the best trainers I know teach women creative ways of building muscle strength without having to purchase weights. Doing push-ups or sit-ups, or working against the resistance of a Dyna-band (available in sporting goods stores) can all be part of such an exercise program.

THE bottom LINE...

Leslie's recommendations for reducing your risk of osteoporosis and bone fracture

1   If you're approaching menopause and deciding whether to take hormone replacement therapy, get your bone density measured to help you and your doctor determine if HRT is required to prevent osteoporosis.

2   If you're already a fan of soy foods, consider boosting your intake so that your diet provides you with 60 to 70 milligrams daily of isoflavones, the natural plant estrogens found in soybeans. Soy's isoflavones bind to estrogen receptors on the bone and may slow down bone loss.

3   To strengthen your bones, make sure you're eating enough protein-rich foods like fish, poultry, lean meat, legumes, tofu, and dairy products. But don't go overboard. Some studies suggest that very high intakes of protein cause your kidneys to excrete calcium.

4   If you drink alcohol, keep your intake at a moderate level of no more than two drinks daily.

5   To prevent too much calcium loss from your body, keep your caffeine intake to a daily maximum of 450 milligrams (that's no more than three small cups of coffee).

6   Go easy on sodium from processed foods and the salt shaker. For every 500 milligrams (1/5 teaspoon) of additional sodium you consume, you need to consume an extra 40 milligrams of calcium to minimize sodium related calcium loss.

7   Depending on your age and your risk for osteoporosis, get 1,000 to 1,500 milligrams of calcium each day from food, and if necessary, supplements.

8   To help you absorb the calcium in your diet, make sure you get 200 to 600 IU of vitamin D each day. The best food sources are fluid milk (not yogurt or cheese), fortified soy or rice beverages, oily fish, and whole eggs. Make a real effort to boost your vitamin D intake in the winter when your body's natural production of the vitamin is reduced by a lack of sunlight.

9   Other nutrients that help build bone density include vitamin A, vitamin K, magnesium, phosphorus, boron, manganese, zinc, and copper. With the exceptions of vitamin K and phosphorus, you'll also find most of these vitamins and minerals in a multivitamin and mineral formula. Vitamin K is made in the body and phosphorus is widespread in commercial foods.

10   If you don't work out now, begin adding regular exercise to your life. Weight bearing activities like brisk walking, jogging, stair climbing, tennis, soccer, and basketball as well as strength training with weights can stimulate an increase in bone density. If you have health problems or you take certain medications, you should check with your physician before embarking on a regular exercise program.

reducing your risk of heart disease

"When I turned 50, the farthest thing from my mind was having a heart attack. I guess I should have paid more attention. It took a long time to accept the fact that at the age of 59 I suffered my first (and hopefully last) heart attack. Today I eat well, exercise, take vitamins, and feel better than ever before."

9

We tend to view heart disease as a health problem faced by middle-aged men. It's true that clogged arteries and heart attacks generally afflict men 10 years earlier than they do women. The fact that women have this built-in protection from heart disease has led many women to believe they are immune to heart attacks. But the physiological factors that protect women end when the menstruating years are over. In the post-menopausal years, the possibility of heart disease needs to be taken very seriously. With the loss of estrogen that accompanies menopause, a woman's risk of getting heart disease increases fourfold and continues to rise with age. If you're a woman older than 50, it's important to realize that your risk of dying from heart disease has increased significantly in comparison to when you were younger. In fact, heart disease and stroke are the top two killers among adult Canadian women, accounting for 40 percent of all deaths.

As women enter menopause they tend to be more concerned about cancer, especially breast cancer. When I ask them, many of my clients say that breast cancer is the leading cause of death among women. In truth, a woman has only one-quarter the risk of dying from breast cancer as she does of heart disease. Women are more anxious about breast cancer because it strikes at a younger age and it kills a greater number of perimenopausal women than heart disease does. But clearly, heart disease takes a larger toll on Canadian women.

I can't emphasize enough how important it is for women to pay attention to their heart health. Both women and their doctors tend to ignore or overlook symptoms like chest pain, often attributing this and other symptoms to indigestion, stress, or gall bladder problems. As well, women tend to get to a hospital much later after having a heart attack than do men, and they also tend to receive less aggressive therapy. Studies have shown that compared to men, women are more likely to die in the year following their heart attack.[1] This is largely due to the fact that women are older and have more advanced heart disease by the time they are diagnosed. As a result, women must learn how to protect themselves from heart disease.

If you're a post-menopausal woman, do not underestimate any chest pain. If heart disease is responsible for your symptoms, the sooner you seek medical attention, the greater your chances of preventing a heart attack. Or, if you experience the warning signs of a heart attack, the sooner you get yourself to an emergency room, the better your recovery will be.

WARNING SIGNS OF A HEART ATTACK

If you experience any of these symptoms, seek medical help immediately.

- Heavy feeling or pressure in the chest area.
- Shortness of breath.
- Nausea and vomiting.
- Sweating.
- Cold, clammy skin.
- Acute, crushing chest pain.
- Pain that moves to your neck, arms, back, jaw.
- A feeling of fear and anxiety; denial of symptoms.

heart disease defined

The term heart disease is really a general term that includes coronary heart disease, congenital heart disease (those with congenital heart disease are born with it), congestive heart failure, and malfunctioning heart valves. What I am going to focus on is coronary heart disease, a disease that affects the blood vessels that feed the heart. Coronary heart disease is the most common type of heart disease, and at the same time, the most easily preventable through dietary and lifestyle adjustments. Coronary heart disease is caused by atherosclerosis, a gradual process that narrows the heart's arteries and leads to a heart attack. To make things simple, I will use the term heart disease to refer to coronary heart disease.

THE PROCESS OF HEART DISEASE

Believe it or not, atherosclerosis can actually can begin in childhood or adolescence. Even in youth, fatty streaks, which may one day cause heart disease, can appear on the lining of the arteries, the vessels through which the heart pumps blood to the body. The fatty streaks are areas where cholesterol is sticking to the artery lining. As cholesterol accumulates, fatty streaks can actually begin to infiltrate the artery wall. As adults, the question is not whether or not we have these fatty areas on our artery walls, but instead what we can do to prevent them from progressing.

Atherosclerosis starts with an injury to the lining of an artery. An infection or virus, high blood pressure, cigarette smoke, or diabetes may cause this damage. Your body attempts to heal itself, just as it would with any wound. The injured area becomes covered with plaque, which contains cholesterol, white blood cells, and smooth muscle cells. Plaque eventually becomes covered with a layer of muscle cells and calcium. As you can see, plaque stiffens arteries and narrows the passage through them. Most people have well developed plaques by the time they're 30.

Atherosclerosis is dangerous because it can restrict blood flow to the heart. Healthy arteries expand with each heartbeat to allow blood to flow easily through them. Once arteries become stiff and narrow from a build-up of plaque, they cannot expand and blood pressure rises. High blood pressure damages the vessel walls further and more plaque forms. As less blood flows through narrowed arteries, your kidneys respond by causing your body to hold on to sodium, which increases your blood pressure further.

HOW A HEART ATTACK HAPPENS

Blood cells called platelets respond to damaged spots on blood vessels by forming clots. Your body uses the same process to form a scab on a cut. Normally clots dissolve in the blood. But when atherosclerosis is severe enough, clots form faster than they can disappear. A clot may stick to plaque and gradually enlarge until it blocks blood flow to an area of the heart. That portion of the heart may die slowly and form scar tissue.

But a clot may also break loose, and circulate in the blood until it reaches an artery too small to pass through. When a clot that's wedged in a vessel cuts off the supply of oxygen and nutrients to a part of the heart muscle, a heart attack results (a stroke occurs when a clot blocks an artery that leads to the brain and kills an area of brain tissue).

risk factors for heart disease

Knowing your risk factors for heart disease is an important first step in reducing your risk. At least half of all heart attacks are the result of known risk factors. The check-list below gives the most important risk factors for heart disease. As you can see, risk factors are classified as either "modifiable" or "non-modifiable." Non-modifiable factors—like your age, or having a family history of early heart attacks—are risk factors that you can't change. Where you exert your control over heart disease is with modifiable risk factors. Culprits like poor diet, lack of exercise, or tobacco use you can eliminate from your life. Others, such as high blood pressure or diabetes, you can control.

Are you at risk for heart disease? Assess your heart health by reviewing the risk factors below. If one or more "modifiable" risk factors apply to you, take action to change these and lower your odds of heart disease.

Non-modifiable risk factors
- You're older than 40.
- You're at or past menopause.
- You have a family history of heart attack prior to age 60.

Modifiable risk factors
- You have high blood cholesterol—or you don't know your blood cholesterol levels.
- You have high blood triglycerides—or you don't know your triglyceride levels.
- You have low HDL cholesterol—or you don't know your HDL levels.
- You have high blood pressure—or you don't know what your blood pressure is.
- You smoke cigarettes.
- You have a poor diet (for example, you eat higher fat foods often and/or your diet is lacking in fruits and vegetables).

- You don't exercise regularly.
- You have diabetes.
- Your BMI is more than 25 (see page 78).

The more heart disease risk factors you have, the higher your risk of developing it. While 62 percent of Canadian women have at least one risk factor for heart disease, 19 percent have at least two, including regular smoking, high blood pressure, or high blood cholesterol. Women who are between the ages of 65 and 74 are most likely to have multiple risk factors. Even small increases in more than one factor can impact your chances of getting the disease. Here's a closer look at the risk factors and how they speed up heart disease.

ADVANCING AGE

As you get older your chances of having heart disease increase. With age, your body becomes less efficient at clearing cholesterol from the bloodstream. The cells in the lining of your blood vessels contain receptors for low density lipoprotein (LDL), a substance that carries cholesterol particles (more on this below). These receptors attach to LDL and remove the cholesterol it carries from the blood. As the adult years pass, your body produces fewer of these receptors and the ones you do have become sluggish. Most of the age-related rise in blood cholesterol occurs between the ages of 20 and 50. This is also a time when many people gain weight and this also accounts for some of the rise in blood cholesterol that occurs during adulthood. With advancing age many women develop high blood pressure and diabetes, two other important risk factors for heart disease.

ONSET OF MENOPAUSE

I mentioned earlier that women get heart disease 10 to 15 years later than men, a fact often referred to as "gender protection." Sometime between the ages of 50 and 55 a woman's estrogen levels decline, and her heart disease risk begins to rise. In men, by contrast, the risk of heart disease increases around the age of 40. Both natural and surgical menopause is associated with an increased risk. Before menopause, estrogen protects the heart by keeping cholesterol levels in check. It does this by stimulating the production of LDL receptors on cell surfaces. The more LDL receptors you have, the more cholesterol can leave the blood and enter the cells where it will be broken down.

With a loss of estrogen, LDL receptor activity declines and blood cholesterol levels rise. Before menopause, estrogen may also help keep blood vessels more flexible.

FAMILY HISTORY

If you have a first degree relative with heart disease you carry a higher risk of getting the disease yourself. As a woman, your risk is even greater if you have a female relative who suffered heart disease. Genes can make you more prone to having high cholesterol, to having LDL cholesterol that's susceptible to free radical damage, or to sustaining an injury to your artery lining. (For more on free radicals, see "Antioxidants: Disease Fighters of the New Millenium" on page 145). Scientists have yet to sort out how your genetic makeup contributes to heart disease. Just keep in mind that a family history doesn't mean you'll get the disease. It means you have a tendency. As you'll see below, there are plenty of positive things you can do so that heart disease has less chance of becoming your destiny.

HIGH BLOOD LIPID LEVELS

By now I'm sure you've heard plenty about high cholesterol levels and heart disease. The strong link between the two is certainly the reason we jumped on the low fat bandwagon in the 1980s. Back then, it was clear that a one percent lowering of blood cholesterol translated into a two percent reduction in heart disease (and as you'll read later, one of the key strategies for lowering high cholesterol levels is to cut back on animal fat).

Nevertheless, many people are still confused about cholesterol. Let me begin by telling you there are two different kinds of cholesterol. Dietary cholesterol is found in foods and blood cholesterol is made by your liver. For most people, the two are unrelated. That means that dietary cholesterol intake has little or no effect on the amount of cholesterol in the blood.

Cholesterol and another type of blood fat made in your liver, the triglycerides, don't dissolve in your blood. That means they have to be transported in the blood piggyback style, on protein carriers (lipoproteins), to their cellular destinations. The lipoproteins that have received the most attention are low density lipoproteins (LDLs) and high density lipoproteins (HDLs). If you've heard these terms used by your doctor, but were never sure what they meant, here's a primer on blood fats.

LDL cholesterol

This cholesterol is transported to the arteries on low density lipoproteins (lipid, or fat carrying proteins). LDL cholesterol is the type that contributes to the process of hardening and narrowing of the arteries. LDL receptor sites in blood vessel walls degrade this type of cholesterol, taking it out of the blood. The potential problems caused by LDL increase when, as explained above, LDL receptor sites decline in number with age. LDL is also more likely to stick to artery walls if it has been damaged by free radicals. The higher your LDL cholesterol levels, the greater your risk of developing heart disease. LDL levels are strongly influenced by what you eat.

HDL cholesterol

High density lipoproteins carry cholesterol away from the arteries towards the liver for degradation. HDLs therefore help prevent the accumulation of cholesterol on your artery walls. The higher your HDL levels, the lower your risk of developing heart disease. HDL levels are influenced by genetics, exercise, and to some extent, diet.

Triglycerides

These fat particles are made in the liver from the food you eat and are transported in your blood on very low density lipoproteins (VLDLs). Although they have not received as much attention as cholesterol, high levels of triglycerides are also associated with a greater risk of heart disease, especially in women over 50. Triglyceride levels are affected by diet, exercise, and weight.

If you know your cholesterol and triglyceride levels, use the following reference guide to find out if your levels are healthy or if they put you at higher risk for heart disease. (Blood lipids are measured in millimoles per litre.)

BLOOD LIPID LEVELS: UNDERSTANDING YOUR RISK

Blood Lipid	Desirable	Borderline Risk	At Risk
Total Cholesterol	< 5.2	5.2–6.2	>6.2
LDL cholesterol	2.0–3.4		>3.4
HDL cholesterol	0.9–2.4		<0.9
Triglycerides	0.6–2.3		>2.3

Circulating cholesterol contributes to heart disease by becoming part of the fatty plaques that build up on artery walls. The more LDL cholesterol there is in the blood, the more cholesterol is available for attachment to artery walls. (As mentioned above, HDL cholesterol, on the other hand, is transported to the liver for excretion.) The longer you have high LDL levels, the greater the chance more cholesterol has built up in your arteries. Now while high LDL cholesterol levels stress your arteries, oxidized LDL cholesterol creates even worse problems. Once LDL cholesterol becomes oxidized, that is, damaged by harmful free radical molecules, it then is much more likely to accumulate in your artery linings. You'll see that my recommendations to prevent heart disease include not only dietary strategies to lower cholesterol, but also ways to protect your LDL cholesterol from oxidation (and you probably can guess that that's where antioxidants play a role!).

ANTIOXIDANTS: DISEASE FIGHTERS OF THE NEW MILLENNIUM

The role dietary antioxidants play in disease prevention has been one of the most important discoveries made in the field of nutrition. Current knowledge indicates that many degenerative diseases (heart disease, cancer, and Alzheimer's, to name just a few) have their origins in free radical damage.

Free radicals are highly reactive oxygen molecules. They are produced by normal body processes, and come into the body from the environment. The reason they are so reactive is that they are missing an electron—most molecules have equal numbers of protons (positively charged particles) and electrons (negatively charged particles). In an effort to restore balance, free radicals seek out electrons from molecules found in body cells and in the process, destroy those cells. The body produces substances that keep free radical activity in check, but levels decline with age. Also, large numbers of environmental free radicals from pollution, cigarette smoke, and the like can overwhelm our natural defenses.

Unchecked free radical activity can damage many components of cells including DNA, lipids (fats), and proteins. One contributing factor to heart disease is free radical damage (oxidation) to LDL cholesterol. Once oxidized, LDL cholesterol is more likely to be deposited on artery walls, where it causes hardening and narrowing of the arteries.

As mentioned above, our bodies are equipped with built-in antioxidant enzymes that search out and neutralize free radicals. Over the past decade, we have also learned that a continual supply of dietary antioxidants is necessary for disease prevention.

Dietary antioxidants include vitamins C and E, beta-carotene, and selenium. And as you read Chapters 9 and 10, you'll discover that there are other protective antioxidant compounds in plant foods as well. You'll learn that eating plenty of fruit, vegetables, and whole grains and adding certain antioxidant supplements to your diet are smart health protection strategies.

Blood cholesterol levels rise quickly in women after menopause. According to Canadian surveys, by the age of 55 women have higher cholesterol levels than men. In fact, 43 percent of Canadian women have a total cholesterol level above 5.2 millimoles per litre and almost one-third have high LDL levels. It seems that having high total cholesterol does not pose as much risk for women as it does for men. What's worse, according to specialists, is having both a low HDL cholesterol level and a high triglyceride level. This combination increases a woman's risk of heart disease by a factor of ten.[2]

In order to get a more accurate picture of your risk for heart disease then, it's important to get *all* types of cholesterol measured, not just your total number. If your total cholesterol is 6.5, but your HDL is high, then your risk for heart disease is lessened. If, on the other hand, your doctor determines that a high LDL level accounts for most of your total value of 6.5 and at the same time your HDL is low, this would be cause for concern. You'd want to make some lifestyle changes to change the numbers for the better.

Recent research also suggests that your ratio of total cholesterol to HDL cholesterol is a better predictor of heart disease risk than LDL or HDL values alone.[3] This number is referred to as your "risk ratio." Here's a guide to this ratio as it applies to women.

TOTAL CHOLESTEROL/HDL CHOLESTEROL (RISK RATIO)

Below average risk	<3.5
Average risk	3.5–5.0
Above average risk	5–10
Much above average risk	>10

HIGH BLOOD PRESSURE

Elevated blood pressure, or hypertension, is considered one of the "big three" risk factors for heart disease (along with high cholesterol and cigarette smoking). The higher blood pressure is above normal, the greater the risk. If your arteries are stiff from atherosclerosis, they strain as blood pulses through them. Add high blood pressure to the equation, and your arteries are put under much greater stress. Stressed and strained arteries develop more lesions and fatty plaque grows more frequently. And as I explained earlier, if you already have hypertension, atherosclerosis makes your high blood pressure worse. If hardened arteries can't expand when the heart beats, then pressure rises. This, in turn, leads to further damage to the arteries. And when blood flow to the kidneys slows down, these organs respond by raising the pressure more through retention of sodium, since from their point of view, blood pressure is too low. Atherosclerosis and high blood pressure can be a deadly combination.

Blood pressure is created by the pressure generated by your heart as it pushes blood through your arteries. When your heart beats, the blood pressure in your arteries rises. When the heart relaxes between beats, blood pressure falls. Your blood pressure is taken with two measures, called systolic pressure (the blood pressure when the heart is contracting) and diastolic pressure (the blood pressure when the heart is relaxing). Hypertension is defined as sustained high blood pressure; usually the systolic reading is over 140 and the diastolic reading is above 90. Doctors usually focus on the diastolic blood pressure to diagnose high blood pressure. Here are the standards used.

DIASTOLIC BLOOD PRESSURE

<85	Normal
80 to 89	High-normal
90 to 99	Mild hypertension
100 to 109	Moderate hypertension
109 to 119	Severe hypertension
≥120	Very severe hypertension

Over one-third of post-menopausal women in Canada have high blood pressure. In fact, after the age of 55, hypertension is more common in women than it is in men. High blood pressure has no symptoms. The only way you can find out if you have high blood pressure is to have your blood pressure checked regularly. Then you can take steps to manage it and minimize the damage it can do to your heart. Your blood pressure should be taken when you are relaxed, not stressed. Many of my clients have gone to their doctor, had their blood pressure measured, and come out with a high reading. Yet two days later, when they are retested, their blood pressure is normal. This phenomenon is often referred to as "white coat syndrome." When you're anxious (and many of us are at medical check-ups) your blood pressure rises. But when you relax it returns to normal. That's why it's also a good idea to have your doctor take a few readings in a row. Chances are, after the first two tests, you'll begin to relax and your doctor will get a more accurate reading.

High blood pressure is treated by weight loss, dietary modifications, and often, medication. Further on in this chapter, you'll find the latest on dietary strategies that help lower high blood pressure.

CIGARETTE SMOKING

It's been estimated that smoking triples a person's risk of developing heart disease. Smoking damages the lining of the arteries, increasing the likelihood of plaque formation. Inhaling cigarette smoke also produces free radicals in the body which then damage LDL cholesterol, making it stick to the artery walls. If that weren't enough, smoking also increases blood pressure and makes blood clot formation more likely.

Among women, smoking is the number one preventable risk factor for heart disease. Interestingly, smoking is a more important predictor of heart attack in middle-aged women than it is in men. And the longer you smoke the greater your chances of heart disease. In the well-known Nurses' Health Study done by Harvard researchers, it was found that women who started smoking before the age of fifteen had a ninefold higher risk of heart disease than women who had never smoked. If you smoke, the sooner you quit the better. The same study found that your risk of dying from heart disease decreases to the risk level of a non-smoker 10 to 14 years after you quit.[4]

Women who use estrogen and smoke cigarettes have an even higher risk because this combination increases the possibility that blood clots will form. If you take birth control pills or hormone replacement therapy and you smoke, seriously consider quitting.

DIABETES

Diabetes, a disease in which blood sugar levels persist at high levels, increases the risk of dying from heart disease more in women than it does in men. A woman with diabetes is three times more likely to experience heart disease than a non-diabetic woman.[5] In fact, if a woman develops diabetes before menopause, her built-in gender protection is gone. The development of fatty plaque progresses much more rapidly in diabetes. Women with diabetes also tend to have abnormal blood lipids (high LDL, low HDL, and high triglyceride levels) and high blood pressure. These three risk factors—diabetes, abnormal blood lipid levels, and high blood pressure—act synergistically to increase heart disease risk and are known collectively as Syndrome X.

WEIGHT

As your body mass index (BMI) increases, so does your risk for heart disease. Carrying extra weight puts stress on your heart and circulatory system. Your heart has to work harder to pump blood throughout your body. Being overweight can also lead to high blood pressure and elevated blood cholesterol. Health Canada estimates that 41 percent of Canadian women are overweight, as they have a BMI over 25; 27 percent are classified as obese, as they have a BMI over 27.[6] To calculate your BMI turn to page 78.

Carrying excess weight around the waist is much more dangerous to your heart than having chunky thighs. In fact, the famous Nurses' Health Study found that women with a waist to hip ratio (WHR) of 0.74 or higher had a twofold increase in heart disease risk.[7] (To determine your WHR see page 78.) According to the Nurses' Health Study an ideal WHR is less than 0.72. Abdominal fat appears to be more active than lower body fat. And when fat stores in this area are mobilized, they go directly to the liver where they are packed into LDL molecules. Researchers are also learning that fat around the middle interferes with blood sugar and insulin levels and can increase the risk of diabetes.

HOMOCYSTEINE LEVELS

Scientists are now turning their attention to a compound called homocysteine. A high blood level of homocysteine is present in 47 percent of people who have early heart disease that can't be explained by other risk factors. Evidence for the role of homocysteine in heart disease has been mounting since 1985 when a paper in the *New England Journal of*

Medicine reported that 30 percent of people with premature heart attack had high blood levels of homocysteine. Since then a number of studies have discovered that people with high homocysteine levels have a much higher risk of developing heart disease than those with normal levels. Recently, American researchers from Boston found that among 28,263 post-menopausal women, those with the highest levels of homocysteine had more than double the risk of heart attack or stroke than women with the lowest levels.[8]

Homocysteine is an amino acid that our body produces naturally in the course of daily biochemical activities. Normally we convert homocysteine to other harmless amino acids with the help of B vitamins. When this conversion doesn't occur, homocysteine can accumulate in the blood and damage vessel walls, promoting the build-up of cholesterol. Homocysteine levels can accumulate as the result of either an inherited genetic defect or a B vitamin deficiency.

Unfortunately you can't just walk into your doctor's office and ask to have your homocysteine levels measured. Not yet anyway. The blood test isn't covered by any of Canada's provincial health insurance plans, and costs anywhere from $30 to $100, depending on where you live. Even at a price, it's not routinely available in hospitals, and the average physician may be unfamiliar with its implications since no clear definition of normal or healthy homocysteine levels has been established yet. But according to some experts in the field of heart disease, a blood test for homocysteine levels may be "standard care" in the near future. If you're left wondering what to do, keep reading to learn what nutrition tips can keep your homocysteine level healthy.

INACTIVITY

Leading a sedentary lifestyle is considered an independent risk factor for heart disease. That means that even if you are free of all the other risk factors, if you don't exercise regularly you're at a higher risk for heart disease. I'm sure you've heard health professionals promote the many benefits of exercise. For starters, regular exercise helps you maintain a healthy weight. Regular aerobic exercise can lower LDL cholesterol levels and raise those of HDL cholesterol. It also strengthens the heart and blood vessels. And there's no doubt in my mind that when people exercise regularly, they tend to make healthier food choices.

I am sure it is apparent by now that you can alter or eliminate many of the risk factors discussed above. Clearly, changing your lifestyle can have a significant impact on your risk for heart disease. According to a recent survey done by the Heart and Stroke Foundation, Canadian women are getting a failing grade when it comes to protecting their future heart health. Up to two-thirds of women are making lifestyle choices that put them at risk—only 30 percent maintain a healthy weight, 36 percent are physically inactive, and only about one-half have talked to their doctor about their risk of heart disease.[9]

The good news is that each one of us has the ability to do something about this situation. Many of the risk factors we've been considering are influenced by what you eat. I think doctors often forget this fact. I can't tell you how many clients come to see me to avoid going on cholesterol lowering medication recommended by their doctor. Their blood tests come back high and the physician hands them a prescription instead of sending them to a nutritionist. Luckily, I work with a number of wonderful physicians who always send their patients my way before resorting to cholesterol lowering drugs!

So now it's time to take a look at what you can do to reduce your odds for heart disease. The strategies I list below will help in a number of ways. My nutrition and herbal recommendations will help to keep your blood lipids at a healthy level, prevent damage or oxidation to your LDL cholesterol, lower blood pressure, and promote a little weight loss. So let's get started!

Dietary approaches

DIETARY FAT

One of the most important strategies for eating "heart healthy" is to reduce your fat intake to less than 30 percent of your total calorie intake. If you're eating a 2,000-calorie diet, that translates into no more than 65 grams of fat per day. If you're following a 1,200-calorie weight loss diet, that means consuming no more than 40 grams of fat per day. You also need to remember that when it comes to heart health, not all fats are created equal. Some fats have a strong impact on your risk, whereas others are neutral, and don't affect your heart. There's no question that nutrition recommendations on types and amounts of dietary fat can be very confusing. To help clear up this confusion once and for all, here's what you need to know about fat to reduce your risk for heart disease.

Saturated fat

This type of fat is found in animal foods—that means it's found in meat, poultry, eggs, and all dairy products. Without a doubt, diets that contain a lot of saturated fat raise your risk for heart disease. Many studies have shown that high intakes of saturated fat are linked with high levels of blood cholesterol. Saturated fat seems to inhibit the activity of LDL receptors on cells so that cholesterol accumulates in the bloodstream.[10]

There are many different types of saturated fats in foods and researchers are learning that they don't all influence our blood cholesterol to the same degree. For instance, the saturated fat in dairy products raises cholesterol more than the saturated fat in meat. And you might be pleased to know that the type of saturated fat found in chocolate (called stearic acid) does not raise blood cholesterol levels. Having just told you this, I don't expect you to know the different types of saturated fats in foods. What's most important is to just eat less saturated fat. Saturated fat should account for less than 10 percent of your daily calories. Here's how you'll achieve that goal.

LOWER FAT SUBSTITUTES FOR COMMON FOODS

Food	Lower fat choices or substitutes
Milk	Skim, 1% milkfat (MF)
Yogurt	Products with less than 1.5% MF
Cheese	Products with less than 20% MF
Cottage Cheese	Products with 1% MF
Sour Cream	Products with 7% MF or less
Cream	Evaporated 2% or evaporated skim milk
Red meat	Flank steak, inside round, sirloin, eye of round, extra lean ground beef, venison
Pork	Centre cut pork chops, pork tenderloin, pork leg (inside round, roast), baked ham, deli ham, back bacon
Poultry	Skinless chicken breast, turkey breast, ground turkey
Egg, whole	Two egg whites replace one egg; you can buy them right beside the fresh eggs in your grocery store. (See my comment on eggs in the section on dietary cholesterol, page 158.)

Deciphering cheese labels

Have you ever wondered what the number accompanying the statement "% MF" (percent milk fat) means on dairy products? It refers to the amount of fat present in a certain *volume* of milk or *weight* of cheese. For example, 31% MF on a package of cheddar cheese means that there are 31 grams of fat in 100 grams of this cheese. In other words, you're getting 9 grams of fat in a 30 gram (1 oz.) serving. Feta cheese labelled as having 22% MF has 6.5 grams of fat per 30 gram (1 oz.) serving. In the case of fluid milk, fat is measured per 100 millilitres of milk. For example, 1% milk contains one gram of fat per 100 millilitres of milk. That translates into 2.5 grams (less than a teaspoon) in one 8-ounce (250 millilitre) glass.

To eat less saturated fat, look for cheese made with part skim milk (15 to 20% MF) or skim milk (7% MF). Or buy naturally lower fat cheeses like feta and chèvre. Then again, you can always use smaller portions of stronger tasting cheeses.

Making lower fat choices will help you eat less saturated fat. But it's also important to watch your portion sizes of these foods. When you do eat lean meat, be sure your portion size doesn't exceed 3 ounces (90 grams). This way you'll also stay within in your serving recommendations for the entire day (refer to Appendix 1, my "Total Nutrition Plan," for the recommended number of daily servings of each food group).

You might be wondering about butter. It is a concentrated source of saturated fat. If your blood cholesterol levels are normal, there is no reason why you can't include butter in your diet. Just use it sparingly. Even if your blood cholesterol levels are high, you can still use a little butter (if you're doing everything else right to lower your cholesterol, it shouldn't make a difference). Many people have made the switch to margarine because, unlike butter, it is made from vegetable oils that don't raise cholesterol. But before you spread your toast with margarine, there's something you should know about another type of fat.

Trans fat

Chances are you've heard this term before. If not, you might have heard about "hydrogenated fat." Before I explain what trans or hydrogenated fats do to your heart, let me first tell you what they are. Hydrogenation is a chemical process that adds hydrogen atoms to liquid vegetable oils. Hydrogenating vegetable oils make them more solid and more useful to food manufacturers. Cookies, crackers, pastries, and muffins made with hydrogenated vegetable oils are more palatable and have a longer shelf life. A margarine that's made by hydrogenating a vegetable oil is firm like butter.

Sounds okay so far. The bad news is that hydrogenation makes a fat become saturated *and* it forms significant amounts of new type of fat called *trans fat* (not to mention the fact that hydrogenation destroys essential fatty acids that we need to obtain from the vegetable oils we eat). Trans fat increases LDL cholesterol and decreases HDL cholesterol levels. Remember that for heart health, we want lower LDL and higher HDL levels. In fact, many researchers believe that trans fat is worse for our cholesterol levels than saturated fat. Harvard researchers have estimated that replacing 2 percent of daily calories from trans fat with a monounsaturated fat like olive oil can reduce the risk of heart disease in women by 53 percent. The Nurses' Health Study revealed that women who had the highest intake of trans fat had a 50 percent higher risk of heart disease than women who ate the least. Foods that contributed to trans fat intake were margarine, cookies, cake, and white bread. An Italian study found similar results. Women who had a medium or high intake of margarine had a 50 percent higher risk of heart attack than those who had a low intake.[11]

The easiest way to reduce your intake of trans fat is to start reading food labels and ingredient lists.

- Look for the words "partially hydrogenated vegetable oils." Eat foods that contain them less often. As much as 40 percent of the fat in foods like French fries, fast food, doughnuts, pastries, snack foods, and commercial cookies is trans fat.

- If you eat margarine, choose one that's made with "non-hydrogenated" fat. Many brands state that they are made of non-hydrogenated fat right on the top label. If you can't see this statement on your tub of margarine, use the nutrition information panel to add up the amounts of polyunsaturated and monounsaturated fats in the margarine. You should arrive at a total of at least six grams per serving. If you don't that means there are more saturated and trans fats present. Time for a brand change!

- You won't find grams of trans fat listed on nutrition labels. But there is one way to tell if trans fats are present. Look at the nutrition information panel and add up the grams of saturated, polyunsaturated, and monounsaturated fat. Compare this number to the total grams of fat figure given. You may find that these numbers don't match—the total fat grams listed may be more than what you get by adding up the individual types of fat. The missing fat grams are trans fat!

NUTRITION TIP

Detecting trans fat

Below are the values found on the nutrition information label of a popular low fat cracker brand. Add up the grams of saturated, polyunsaturated, and monounsaturated fat. Compare this number to the total grams of fat given on the label. You may find that these numbers don't match—the total fat grams listed may be more than what you get by adding up the individual types of fat. The missing fat grams are trans fat! Do these crackers contain trans fat? How much?

Nutrition Information

1 Serving = 20 g = Approx. 15 crackers

Per Serving

Energy	91 Cal
	380 kJ
Protein	1.1 g
Fat	2.9 g
Polyunsaturates	0.1 g
Monounsaturates	1.4 g
Saturates	0.5 g
Cholesterol	0 mg
Carbohydrate	15 g

You see there's almost one gram of fat per serving unaccounted for!

Polyunsaturated fat

These fats are classified by scientists according to their chemical structure. Omega-6 polyunsaturated fats are found in all vegetable oils including canola, sunflower, safflower, corn, and sesame. Omega-3 polyunsaturates are found in fish and seafood, and flaxseed and walnut oil. Replacing saturated fat in your diet with polyunsaturated fats has a cholesterol lowering effect. For instance, using a non-hydrogenated margarine made from sunflower oil instead of butter, or eating fish instead of steak are ways to reduce high blood cholesterol levels. Most of this effect is due to the fact that you are eating less saturated fat, not because the polyunsaturated fats have magical properties. In fact, animal studies have found that adding polyunsaturated fat to the diet while keeping the amount of saturated fat constant does not result in cholesterol reduction.[12]

Fish and heart health   It does seem, however, that there is something special about the polyunsaturated fat in fish. Omega-3 fats from fish can lower high levels of triglycerides and reduce the stickiness of platelets, the cells that form blood clots in arteries. Omega-3s may also increase the flexibility of red blood cells so that they can pass more readily through tiny blood vessels. Many studies have found that populations who consume fish a few times each week have lower rates of heart disease.[13]

How much fish should you eat? The Canadian Heart and Stroke Foundation makes no specific recommendations about fish consumption, but most experts agree we should eat fish three times a week to reap the beneficial effects of omega-3 fats. For more omega-3s choose oilier fish—salmon, trout, sardines, herring, mackerel, swordfish, and fresh tuna are good choices. If you plan to rely on tuna fish sandwiches to get your omega-3s, think twice. Canned tuna has very little heart healthy oil!

Flaxseed, canola, and walnut oils   Still on the subject of polyunsaturated fats, we also need to take into account that the only way we can meet our need for the two essential fatty acids, alpha-linolenic acid (ALA) and linoleic acid (LA) is to eat certain polyunsaturated fats. ALA and LA are needed to produce prostaglandins, hormone-like substances that regulate many aspects of our functioning. ALA is found in canola, walnut, and flaxseed oils and may help prevent heart disease. In a study of almost 77,000 women, those who consumed the most ALA had a 45 percent lower risk of dying from heart disease.[14] When the investigators looked at what these women were eating, they found that a higher intake of oil and vinegar salad dressing accounted for the ALA in their diet. The women who used vinaigrette salad dressings at least five or six times a week reduced their risk of dying from heart disease by 54 percent. The message here—a little fat is necessary for heart health. Don't be tempted to avoid oils altogether. If you choose the right ones, and use them sparingly, you just might ward off heart disease.

Monounsaturated fat

Monounsaturated fats found in olive oil, canola oil, and peanut oil are considered to be neutral with respect to cholesterol levels. That is, they don't influence blood cholesterol levels on their own. But when you substitute them for saturated fat, you can lower high levels of blood cholesterol. But as is the case with polyunsaturated fat, that's because you're cutting back on saturated fat. Monounsaturated fats are certainly good fats to include in the diet though. Some studies suggest that extra virgin olive oil helps prevent blood clots from forming and has antioxidant effects that help protect its users from heart disease.[15] If you do use olive oil, be sure to buy the extra virgin type that's darker in colour. I know it's more expensive, but it has been processed the least and contains more protective compounds. But remember—don't overdo it with olive oil. Whether it's olive oil, margarine, or butter it still has 9 calories per gram. Too much of any type of fat can cause weight gain, and this in turn can increase your blood cholesterol levels. To follow a low fat diet, you should aim to consume no more than one or two tablespoons (15 to 30 millilitres) of added fat each day.

RESEARCH FILE

The Mediterranean diet and heart health

If Greek or Italian foods are your favourite fare, you might be interested to know that these cuisines can protect your heart. Recently, researchers compared the effects of the Mediterranean diet to those of the typical western diet in 423 people who had experienced one heart attack. After 27 months, the Mediterranean diet showed striking protective effects. Heart disease related death rates and heart attack recurrences were much lower in those who followed the Mediterranean diet, rich in fruit, vegetables, grains, beans, olive oil and fish.[16]

Follow the guidelines below to save the airfare to Italy and reap the health benefits of this diet!

Daily foods

- Rice, pasta, couscous, breads
- Fruits and vegetables
- Legumes (lentils, kidney beans, chickpeas)
- Extra virgin first cold pressed olive oil
- Yogurt and cheese

A few times a week
- Fish, chicken, eggs
- Sweets

A few times a month
- Red meat

Dietary cholesterol

This wax-like fatty substance is found in meat, poultry, eggs, dairy products, fish, and seafood. It's particularly plentiful in shrimp, liver, and egg yolks. While high cholesterol diets cause high blood cholesterol in animals, this effect is not seen in humans. In fact, dietary cholesterol has little or no effect on most people's blood cholesterol. One reason for this is that our intestines absorb roughly one-half of the cholesterol we eat. The rest is excreted in the stool. Our bodies are also very efficient at secreting the cholesterol we do absorb from food into bile that's stored in the gall bladder. What this means is that very little dietary cholesterol becomes available for transport on LDL particles. So if you're worried about eating eggs, you need not be. A recent study done at Harvard University did not find any significant association between egg intake and risk of heart disease or stroke in healthy men and women.[17] Most experts agree that eating five or six eggs a week will not negatively affect your heart health.

In spite of these built-in protective mechanisms, too much dietary cholesterol can raise LDL cholesterol levels in some people, especially people with a hereditary predisposition to high cholesterol. Health Canada recommends that we consume no more than 300 milligrams of cholesterol each day. Choosing animal foods that are lower in saturated fat also helps to cut down on dietary cholesterol. Here's how foods stack up when it comes to cholesterol content.

CHOLESTEROL CONTENT OF COMMON FOODS (MILLIGRAMS)

1 egg, whole	216
1 egg, white only	0
Beef sirloin, lean only, 3 oz. (90 g)	64
Calf's liver, fried, 3 oz. (90 g)	416
Pork loin, lean only, 3 oz. (90 g)	71
Chicken breast, no skin, 3 oz. (90 g)	73

Salmon, 3 oz. (90 g)	54
Shrimp, 3 oz. (90 g)	135
Milk, 2% MF, 1 cup (250 ml)	19
Milk, skim, 1 cup (250 ml)	5
Cheese, cheddar, 31% MF, 1 oz. (30 g)	31
Cheese, mozzarella, part skim, 1 oz. (30 g)	18
Cream, half and half, 12% MF, 2 tbsp. (25 ml)	12
Yogurt, 1.5% MF, 3/4 cup (175 ml)	11
Butter, 2 tsp. (10 ml)	10

SOY PROTEIN

It's clear that a daily dose of soy lowers blood cholesterol. So clear, in fact, that in October 1999 the U.S. Food and Drug Administration passed a regulation allowing manufacturers of soy foods to add a health claim on the label. Cartons of tofu, soy beverages, and veggie burgers now tell American shoppers that eating a low fat diet containing 25 grams of soy protein daily lowers the risk for heart disease.

The soy and heart disease link became popular knowledge back in 1995 when researchers from Lexington, Kentucky published a report in the *New England Journal of Medicine* that analyzed 38 studies on soy and cholesterol. The analysis determined that eating soy protein instead of animal protein significantly lowered high levels of LDL cholesterol and triglycerides. Since that time, other studies have confirmed soy's cholesterol lowering power. One study showed that 20 grams of soy protein taken daily significantly lowered cholesterol levels in 53 perimenopausal women who had *normal* cholesterol levels to begin with. Another study found that a high soy diet lowered LDL cholesterol by four percent in people with mildly elevated cholesterol levels. This same study found the effect of soy to be even more pronounced in participants with higher cholesterol levels. In these people, LDL cholesterol levels dropped by 10 percent.

Soy can keep your heart healthy in other ways too. Studies show that soy raises HDL cholesterol levels, lowers blood pressure, and keeps blood vessels healthy. Soy also prevents oxidation or damage to LDL cholesterol. As discussed above, when LDL becomes damaged by free radicals, it then sticks to artery walls much more easily. In one study, American researchers found that post-menopausal women who consumed three glasses of soy beverage each day experienced a significant delay in oxidation of LDL cholesterol.[18]

The heart protective effects of soy foods are attributed to the proteins and isoflavones (phytoestrogens) found in soybeans. When it comes to lowering cholesterol levels, you need both components. That's why studies using purified soy based isoflavone supplements don't show a cholesterol lowering effect. If you want to keep your LDL cholesterol levels healthy, I recommend that you add 25 grams of soy protein to your low fat diet each day. Make your plans armed with the following information:

SOY PROTEIN CONTENT OF SOY FOODS (GRAMS)

Soy beverage, I cup (250 ml)	9
Soybeans, canned, 1/2 cup (125 ml)	14
Soy nuts, 1/4 cup (50 ml)	14
Soy flour, defatted, 1/4 cup (50 ml)	13
Soy protein powder, isolate, I scoop (30g)	25
Tempeh, 1/2 cup (125 ml)	16
Tofu, firm, 1/2 cup (125 ml)	19
Tofu, regular, 1/2 cup (125 ml)	10
Veggie burger, Yves Veggie Cuisine, I	11
Veggie dog, small, Yves Veggie Cuisine, I	11

SOLUBLE FIBRE

Plant foods contain a mixture of two types of fibre, soluble and insoluble. While they are both important to your health, it's soluble fibre that can help keep your heart healthy (insoluble fibre found in wheat bran and other plant foods helps keep your bowels healthy). Soluble fibre consists of plant components that either dissolve or swell in water. In plants, soluble fibres help "glue" cells together. The best food sources of these fibres include oats and oat bran, psyllium, legumes or beans, fruits, and vegetables.

Strong evidence exists to support the idea that adding soluble fibre from oats and beans to your low fat diet significantly lowers total and LDL cholesterol levels. American researchers from Chicago studied 146 adults with high LDL cholesterol and found that adding oatmeal and oat bran to a low fat diet lowered LDL cholesterol levels by 10 and 16 percent repsectively.

Psyllium is another type of soluble fibre with cholesterol-lowering effects. An analysis of twelve studies conducted among 404 adults with high cholesterol levels revealed that a pysllium-enriched breakfast cereal, eaten as part of a low fat diet, lowered total cholesterol levels by five percent and LDL cholesterol levels by nine percent.[19]

Based on years of research showing the protective effects of oat fibre (called beta glucan) and pysllium, the U.S. Food and Drug Administration now allows foods rich in these fibres to carry a health claim on their label. Breakfast cereals and other foods that meet specific criteria (high in fibre, low in saturated fat and cholesterol) may state that they help reduce the risk of heart disease in conjunction with a low fat diet (just like foods rich in soy protein).

Soluble fibre actually exerts its cholesterol lowering effect in your intestinal tract. When these fibres reach your intestines, they attach themselves to bile acids and cause these to be excreted in the stool. Bile is a digestive aid that's released from your gall bladder after you eat. Your liver makes bile from cholesterol and sends it to your gall bladder to be stored until it's needed. This means that if a high fibre diet is causing you to excrete more bile, your liver has to make more of it from cholesterol. The end result? Lower blood cholesterol levels. But soluble fibre probably works another way too. When unabsorbed fibre reaches your colon, intestinal bacteria degrade it—short chain fatty acids are byproducts of this bacterial activity. These fatty acids then make their way to the liver where they are able to hamper cholesterol production.

To boost your intake of soluble fibre, here are the foods you'll want to add to your diet:

FOODS HIGH IN SOLUBLE FIBRE

Breakfast Cereals	Legumes	Fruits	Vegetables
Oatmeal	Kidney beans	Orange	Carrots
Oat bran	Black beans	Grapefruit	Potatoes
All Bran Buds	Chickpeas	Apples	Sweet potatoes
Psyllium-enriched cereals	Lentils	Strawberries	Green peas
	Soybeans	Pears	
	Navy beans	Cantaloupe	

If you decide to try a psyllium-rich breakfast cereal, start slowly. These cereals offer a great way to get a hefty dose of soluble fibre and I often encourage my clients with high cholesterol to add them to their breakfast routine. However, they can cause gastrointestinal upset if you're not used to them. As a rule, it takes about two weeks for the bacteria that reside in your intestine to adjust to a higher fibre intake. In the meantime, you may experience bloating and gas. So start by adding 1/4 to 1/2 cup (50 to 125 millilitres) of Bran Buds to your usual cereal. Over the course of two or three weeks, work up to one cup (250 millilitres). And don't forget to drink more water as you increase your fibre intake. Soluble fibre needs fluid in order to do its job!

WHOLE GRAINS

When you think of whole grains, you probably think of fibre. While it's true that foods like whole wheat bread, whole grain breakfast cereals, and brown rice are higher in fibre than their white counterparts, they also have other protective ingredients that might help lower the risk of heart disease.

NUTRITION TIP

Uncommon grains

Need a change from pasta? Bored of rice with your chicken? Maybe it's time to add a little adventure (and nutrition) to your meals with these tasty whole grains.

Buckwheat Probably familiar to many of you as a grain used in pancakes, buckwheat is also sold as kasha and as the main ingredient in Japanese soba noodles. Kasha, sometimes called roasted buckwheat groats, cooks quickly and is very versatile. Try it in soups, stews, stuffing, and stir-fries. It has a nutty taste that boosts the flavour of any meal.

Bulgur If you've eaten Middle Eastern cuisine, chances are you've met bulgur, or cracked whole wheat, in tabouli salad. It's high in iron, calcium, and fibre and great in pilafs, soups, and stuffings. It's another quick cooking grain.

Kamut This grain is related to wheat, but is less likely to cause an allergic reaction. Kamut grains are about two or three times the size of wheat berries and have more fibre and protein than most grains. Kamut's chewy texture and buttery flavour make it great for salads. Commercial food processors grind it into flour used in baked goods, cereals, and pasta.

Quinoa   Sacred to the Incas, this fluffy grain is sold as a whole grain or in pasta form. It's lower in carbohydrate and higher in protein than most grains. Try it in pilafs, salads, casseroles, and stir-fries.

Spelt   Touted, like kamut, as a grain well tolerated by people with wheat allergies, spelt is sold as a whole grain or a flour. You can also buy spelt bread, breakfast cereal, and pasta. Try using the flour in baking and cooking. It adds a delicious nutty taste to pizza crusts and multi-grain breads.

Harvard researchers learned from the Nurses' Health Study that women who had the highest intake of whole grains had a 33 percent lower risk of heart disease than women who consumed the least. Once the researchers accounted for other risk factors like body weight, alcohol intake, and physical activity, whole grains still reduced the risk by 25 percent. Interestingly, whole grains offered the most protection for women who had never smoked—these women had a 52 percent lower risk than smokers. The Iowa Women's Health Study also found a link between whole grain intake and heart health. In this study of almost 35,000 post-menopausal women, those who ate two servings of whole grains each day had the lowest rates of heart disease.[20]

Experts attribute the heart protective effects of whole grains to a number of natural compounds. Whole grains are important sources of vitamin E, minerals such as zinc, selenium, copper, iron, and manganese, and phenolic compounds. All of these natural compounds have antioxidant properties and may offer protection from heart disease. Antioxidants protect your LDL cholesterol from oxidation caused by free radicals. I mentioned earlier that when your LDL cholesterol becomes oxidized, it sticks to artery walls causing a build-up of fatty plaque.

Eating foods made from whole grains means you're getting *all* parts of the grain— the outer bran layer where nearly all the fibre is, the germ layer that's rich in nutrients like vitamin E, and the endosperm that contains the starch. When whole grains are milled, scraped, refined, and heat processed into flakes, puffs, or white flour, all that's left is the starchy endosperm. That means you get significantly less vitamin E, B6, magnesium, potassium, zinc, fibre from these products... the list goes on. Use the following guide to help you get more nutritious whole grains in your diet. I've given you a list of common whole grains and whole grain products, and, where applicable, their refined counterparts.

WHOLE AND REFINED GRAINS

Whole grain	Refined grain
Hulled barley	Pearled barley
Brown rice	White rice
Bulgur	Couscous, semolina, Cream of Wheat
Coarse corn meal or grits	Cornmeal
Flaxseed	
Kamut	
Oatmeal	
Oat Bran	
Quinoa	
Whole wheat bread*	White bread
Whole grain pasta (brown rice, kamut, quinoa, spelt, whole wheat)	Durum semolina or wheat pasta
Whole rye bread	Light rye bread
Spelt	

*When buying bread look for the words "whole wheat flour" on the list of ingredients. The terms "wheat flour" and "unbleached wheat flour" mean that refined wheat flour has been used.

NUTS

It seems that adding a handful of nuts to your diet on a regular basis may also help keep your heart in shape. Populations that include nuts as a regular part of their diet have lower rates of heart disease. The diets of vegetarians, Seventh Day Adventists, Mediterranean, and Asian cultures all include nuts. The Nurses' Health Study discovered that women who ate five ounces of nuts each week had a 35 percent lower risk of heart attack and death from heart disease than women who never ate nuts or ate them less than once a month.

The protective effect of nuts may be due to ingredients similar to those found in whole grains. Nuts and seeds are rich sources of the potent antioxidant vitamin E. They also contain many important minerals. And, of course, nuts are good sources of essential fatty acids (alpha-linolenic acid and linoleic acid) as well as of dietary fibre. A recent French study found that a high level of HDL cholesterol was associated with a diet rich in walnuts.[21]

While researchers determine exactly how nuts work to reduce the risk of heart disease, it makes sense to add them to your diet. Keep your serving size to one ounce (30 grams)—about 1/4 cup (50 millilitres). Aim to get nuts into your diet five times a week. Here's how you might do that:

- Toss a handful of peanuts into an Asian-style stir-fry.
- Nuts are great with greens. Stir-fry collard greens with cashews and a teaspoon (five millilitres) of sesame oil; add walnuts to your green or spinach salad; try a little walnut oil in your next salad dressing (use half olive oil and half walnut oil).
- Mix sunflower or pumpkin seeds into a bowl of hot cereal or yogurt.
- Snack on a small handful of almonds with a few dried apricots.
- Serve your casserole with a sprinkling of mixed nuts.

TEA AND FLAVONOIDS

You've probably never thought of your afternoon cup of orange pekoe as a source of antioxidants that can protect your heart. Well, according to researchers it's true—green and black teas may lower the risk of heart attack. One recent study investigated the effects of tea, coffee, and decaffeinated coffee on heart attack risk. Compared to non-tea drinkers, those who enjoyed at least one cup a day had a 44 percent lower risk of heart attack. In this study, coffee showed no protective (or harmful) effects.

Another study from the Netherlands looked at tea intake in men and women over 55 years old. The researchers found that tea had significant protective effects. The more tea consumed, the lower the risk of atherosclerosis. Drinking one to two cups of tea each day was associated with a 46 percent lower risk of severe atherosclerosis, and drinking more than four cups a day lowered the risk by 60 percent. This study found the protective effect of tea to be stronger in women than men.[22]

Tea leaves contain dietary compounds called flavonoids. Literally hundreds of different flavonoids have been identified in plants and the ones in tea are called catechins. You'll find catechins in green tea, black tea, and oolong tea, but not herbal teas. That's because herbal teas are not made from the leaves of the tea plant, but from the roots, leaves, stems, flowers, and fruits of other plants that do not contain catechins. And a daily cup or two of tea can do more than keep your arteries healthy. In Chapter 10 you'll read about how tea might help reduce your risk of breast cancer too.

The following suggestions will help you incorporate tea into your daily diet:

- Replace that afternoon coffee with a mug of tea.
- Instead of drinking soft drinks, try iced tea. Make your own to avoid the large amounts of sugar found in commercial brands.
- Try different flavours of black tea—Earl Grey, orange spice, apricot, raspberry, and black currant are a few favourites.
- Try a chai latte at your local coffee shop. It's a hot drink made from tea, milk, and spices. Again, these drinks tend to be sweet. Ask for less syrup or sugar than usual to be added.

RESEARCH FILE

Boost your flavonoid intake

If you've starting drinking more tea to get heart protective flavonoids, that's great! But don't stop there. Research suggests you should also be reaching for other foods rich in flavonoids. A study done in the Netherlands found that the risk of dying from heart disease was 48 percent lower in men who had the highest intake of dietary flavonoids (I'm afraid this study didn't look at women). Tea, onions, and apples were the foods rich in flavonoids that appeared to offer these men protection. The Iowa Women's Health Study also found a protective effect from a flavonoid-rich diet. Among these 34,000 post-menopausal women, those who consumed the most flavonoids from food had a 38 percent lower risk of dying from heart disease. In this study, broccoli was strongly linked to a reduced risk.[23] It seems you can't go wrong with plenty of vegetables!

ALCOHOL

Those of you who enjoy a glass of wine with dinner might be doing your heart a favour. Many studies have found that a moderate intake of alcohol reduces the risk of heart disease. The Nurses' Health Study determined that, compared to non-drinkers, women who consumed one to six drinks a week had a 12 to 17 percent lower risk of dying from heart disease. Women who drank more than six drinks a week had a slightly higher risk of death from heart disease.

Scientists believe that alcohol may work in three ways to protect the heart. First, drinking alcohol, whether it's from wine, beer, or liquor, raises the level of HDL cholesterol. A Boston study found that men and women who regularly consumed a few alcoholic drinks had higher levels of HDL cholesterol and a lower risk of heart attack.[24] Second, alcohol may also reduce blood clotting—excessive clotting, as discussed, being part of the process of heart disease. Before you get too excited though, you should know that the protective effects of alcohol are most apparent in people over the age of 50 and in those with more than one risk factor for heart disease. If you're a healthy, premenopausal woman, a daily drink probably won't do much for your heart.

Third, some evidence exists to support the theory that antioxidants in wine, especially red wine, may help keep LDL cholesterol healthy and reduce blood clotting. That's one explanation for the "French Paradox"—people living in France have much lower rates of heart disease than North Americans, despite the fact that they have the same risk factors we do. Some believe that the French are protected by their daily intake of red wine.

Despite the positive research findings, you won't find me advising you to consume a couple of glasses of wine a day. That's because there are too many negative health effects associated with a moderate alcohol intake (one to two drinks daily). For starters, light to moderate drinking increases the risk of breast cancer (Chapter 10 tells you more about this). And if you're suffering through perimenopausal symptoms such as hot flashes, mood swings, and insomnia, alcohol will only make you feel worse. Here's my recommendations regarding alcohol:

- If you drink now, keep your intake to no more than two drinks a day, preferably one.
- If you are a non-drinker don't start now. I believe it's a healthier way to go and as you can see by now, there are plenty of other nutrition strategies you can put in place to reduce the odds of heart disease.

DASH FOR HEALTH

I promised you earlier that I'd give you strategies for lowering high blood pressure. Many of the recommendations already mentioned in this chapter will help to lower elevated blood pressure at the same time as they work to keep your cholesterol levels healthy—eating a low fat diet, drinking alcohol in moderation, and maintaining a healthy weight are all important strategies for keeping blood pressure normal. In addition, there are some other modifications you should consider making to your diet and lifestyle if you want to keep your blood pressure healthy and your risk of heart disease down.

Much of this advice comes from the Dietary Approaches to Stop Hypertension research study, DASH for short, an eight-week trial that measured the effects of diet on blood pressure in 459 adults. Researchers gave participants one of three diets: 1) a control diet that contained low amounts of fruit and vegetables (3.6 servings a day) and dairy products (0.5 servings a day); 2) a diet high in fruits and vegetables (8 to 10 servings a day) and; 3) a combination diet high in fruits and vegetables with added low fat dairy products (2 servings a day). All diets provided the same amounts of sodium and a maximum of two alcoholic drinks per day.

When it came to lowering blood pressure, the combination diet gave the best results. Individuals on this diet who had mild hypertension achieved a reduction in blood pressure similar to that obtained by drug treatment![25] A study is now underway to determine if lowering sodium intake further would make even more of a difference.

If you have high blood pressure and would like to follow the DASH diet, use the following as your guide:

EATING TO LOWER BLOOD PRESSURE

Food group	Number of servings* per day
Whole grain foods	7–8
Vegetables	4–5
Fruits	4–5
Low fat/non fat dairy products	2
Meat, poultry, fish	4–6 oz. (120 to 180 g) or less per day
Legumes, nuts, seeds	4–5
Added fats	3
Sweets	1 serving per week

*For serving size information, refer to Appendix 2, "What's A Serving?"

Here are a few more strategies that will help you maintain healthy blood pressure:
- Don't smoke. Every single cigarette you smoke raises your blood pressure.
- Limit your alcohol intake to no more than two drinks daily.

- Limit sodium intake. To help you see where we get most of our sodium, refer to pages 116–117.
- Get regular exercise. A fitness program of brisk walking can help lower blood pressure.

vitamins and minerals

B VITAMINS

The B vitamins won't lower your cholesterol, but they will help keep your homocysteine level down. I told you earlier that a high level of homocysteine is associated with a higher risk of heart attack. In order to prevent homocysteine from accumulating and damaging blood vessels, the body uses three B vitamins to convert it into other harmless compounds. Folate, vitamin B6, and vitamin B12 are needed for normal homocysteine metabolism—without them, homocysteine levels rise.

One of the simplest strategies for lowering elevated homocysteine levels, then, is to boost your intake of B vitamins. Harvard researchers proved this point when they studied 80,000 women for 14 years and found that those who consumed the most folate and vitamin B6 had a 45 percent lower risk of heart disease than those women who consumed the least.[26] Among those women who got plenty of B vitamins in their diet, the risk of heart disease was also lower if they regularly took a multivitamin and mineral supplement, a major source of folate and B6. Here's how to get more Bs into your daily diet.

FOOD SOURCES OF THE B VITAMINS

B vitamin	RDA	Best food sources
Folate	400 micrograms (0.4 mg)	Spinach, orange juice, lentils, wheat germ, broccoli, leafy greens, whole grains
Vitamin B6	1.3–1.5 mg	Whole grains, bananas, potatoes, legumes, fish, meat, poultry
Vitamin B12	2.4 micrograms	Meat, poultry, fish, dairy products, eggs, fortified soy and rice milk

What about a B vitamin supplement?

I just told you that a daily multiple vitamin offered women in the Nurses' Health Study a little more protection. It's also true that meeting the daily requirement for folate (called folic acid when it's in a supplement) is a challenge for many people. The top three food sources are spinach (262 micrograms per cup—250 millilitres—cooked), lentils (357 micrograms per cup—250 millilitres—cooked), and orange juice (109 micrograms per cup, or 250 millilitres). If you don't eat these foods every day, then you must be sure to eat plenty of other folate-rich foods.

For those of you who have difficulty eating a varied diet, I recommend taking a good quality multivitamin and mineral supplement to ensure you're getting your daily B vitamins. A high quality multivitamin and mineral supplement will provide 100 percent or more of the daily recommended amount of each B vitamin. If you're over 50 you should be getting your B12 from a supplement anyway. That's because as we age, we become less efficient at producing stomach acid, which is necessary for B12 absorption from food. If you're a vegan and don't eat animal foods or fortified beverages, you won't be getting any vitamin B12 from your diet. Yet another reason to take a multivitamin. Use the following criteria when choosing a multivitamin:

- Look for a supplement that offers 0.4 to 1.0 milligrams of folic acid (folate).
- Premenopausal women should look for at least 10 milligrams of iron and preferably 15 milligrams. Post-menopausal women have lower iron requirements and can choose a multi containing 10 milligrams or less.
- A multivitamin/mineral should contain beta carotene, vitamin A, and vitamins D, B1, B2, B6, B12. Biotin and pantothenic acid aren't important since they're easily found in food.
- In terms of minerals, a supplement should contain iron, copper, zinc, magnesium, iodine, selenium, and chromium. Don't worry if you don't see phosphorus or potassium since these are widely distributed in the diet. As for calcium, you can't get enough from a multivitamin. If you need supplemental calcium, you'll have to take that separately.
- Take your supplement with food to allow for better breakdown and absorption of the pill. Plan to take your supplements at the meal you are most likely to remember them.

- If you're looking for more B vitamins than a regular multi gives you, choose a "high potency" formula that contains from 30 to 75 milligrams of most of the B vitamins. One word of caution: the B vitamin niacin may cause flushing of the face and chest when it's taken in doses greater than 35 milligrams (this reaction is easily avoided by taking your supplement at or just after a meal). While this symptom is harmless and goes away within 20 minutes, some people find it uncomfortable. If you want to avoid the flushing response, look for a formula that contains no more than 35 milligrams of niacin. Or choose one containing niacinamide instead, a form of niacin that doesn't cause flushing.

To further boost your B intake, have your multivitamin with a glass of orange juice each morning, order a spinach salad with your whole grain sandwich at lunch, and throw some canned lentils into your pasta sauce at dinner. That doesn't sound so bad does it?

VITAMIN C

Chances are, you're familiar with this vitamin's role in treating the common cold. But you might be surprised to learn that vitamin C could help reduce your risk of a heart attack. Many studies have reported links between high dietary intakes of this vitamin, high blood levels of vitamin C, and a lower risk of heart disease. Finnish scientists measured thirteen risk factors for heart attack in a large group of men and found that low blood levels of vitamin C were the strongest predictor of heart disease. Back home in North America, researchers observed an 11 percent reduction in rates of heart disease with every 0.5 milligram per decilitre rise in blood vitamin C among 6,624 men and women. In fact, in the men and women with the highest blood vitamin C levels, rates of heart disease were 27 percent lower than in those study participants with the lowest vitamin C levels.

It is well accepted that the level of vitamin C in your bloodstream is a good indicator of the amount of vitamin C in your diet. A Portuguese study of 194 adults determined that, compared to those individuals with marginal vitamin C intakes, those who consumed the most vitamin C had an 80 percent lower risk of heart attack.[27]

Vitamin C's claim to fame lies in its ability to act as an antioxidant. The vitamin is able to neutralize harmful free radical molecules that damage your LDL cholesterol (for a more detailed explanation of what free radicals are and how they affect you, read

"Antioxidants: Disease Fighters of the New Millennium" on page 145). As a result, LDL cholesterol is less likely to accumulate on artery walls. But vitamin C may protect your heart in other ways as well. It may raise levels of HDL cholesterol and at the same time, lower LDL cholesterol. And studies suggest the vitamin may also help to inhibit the formation of blood clots by reducing the stickiness of platelets.[28]

The daily recommended vitamin C intake for adult women is 30 milligrams (smokers need double that amount). This amount is easy to get from your diet. Scientists are in the process of revising the daily requirement for C. Studies have shown that higher intakes of this vitamin may help prevent heart disease and certain cancers. In the year 2000, I'm sure we will be told to get at least 100 milligrams each day. So while we wait for new official recommendations, boost your intake of foods rich in this antioxidant vitamin.

NUTRITION TIP

Boosting your C

If your diet needs an infusion of vitamin C, here's a look at your best bets:

CONTENT OF FOODS RICH IN VITAMIN C (MILLIGRAMS)

Cantaloupe, 1/4 medium	56
Orange, 1 medium	70
Orange juice, fresh, 1 cup (250 ml)	131
Grapefruit, red or pink, 1/2	47
Kiwi, 1 large	68
Mango, 1	49
Strawberries, raw, 1 cup (250 ml)	89
Broccoli, raw, 1 spear	141
Brussels sprouts, cooked, 1/2 cup (125 ml)	50
Cauliflower, raw, 1/2 cup (125 ml)	38
Potato, baked with skin, 1	27
Red pepper, raw, 1/2 cup (125 ml)	95
Tomato juice, 1 cup (250 ml)	47

What about Vitamin C supplements?

For those of you who don't eat at least two foods rich in vitamin C each day, a supplement is a good idea. Keep in mind though that fruits and vegetables contain many other natural chemicals that may work together with vitamin C to keep you healthy. So even if you do take a vitamin C pill each day, I recommend that you still try to add foods rich in vitamin C to your diet. Here's what you need to know about vitamin C supplements:

- If you're looking for the most C for your money, choose a supplement labeled "Ester C." Lab studies have found this form of vitamin C to be more available to the body.

- If you don't like to swallow pills and prefer a chewable supplement, make sure it contains calcium ascorbate or sodium ascorbate. These forms of vitamin C are less acidic and corrode your tooth enamel less.

- Take a 500-milligram supplement once or twice a day. There's little point in swallowing much more at one time since your body can only use about 200 milligrams at one time. If you want to take more, split your dose over the day.

VITAMIN E

Data showing that vitamin E protects against coronary heart disease dates back to the 1970s. As scientists began to understand the antioxidant effects of the vitamin, more and more reports emerged suggesting a beneficial cardiovascular effect. Most of the evidence indicates that vitamin E is more effective at preventing heart disease from establishing itself in the first place than it is at treating it. A number of studies have shown that vitamin E supplements prevent heart attacks in men and women. The relationship between vitamin E and the heart was made famous in 1993 by two reports in *The New England Journal of Medicine.* In one of these, a large study of American nurses, women who took supplemental vitamin E (100 international units or IU) for two years had a 41 percent lower risk of heart attack than non-supplement users. In 1996, a Canadian study reported that the use of vitamin supplements, especially of vitamin E, was associated with a reduced risk of heart attack among 2,313 French Canadian men.

Vitamin E may also help prevent a heart attack if you already have atherosclerosis, although the research findings on this question are less consistent. The Cambridge Heart Antioxidant Study gave individuals with heart disease 800 IU or 400 IU of vitamin E daily for one year. The researchers determined that vitamin E use lowered the risk of fatal and non-fatal heart attacks by 47 percent.[29]

Vitamin E is often referred to as the superstar lipid antioxidant. Once consumed, vitamin E makes its way to the liver where it is incorporated into cell membranes and carrier molecules, such as the lipoproteins that transport cholesterol. It is in these carrier molecules that vitamin E works to protect the lipids from damage by free radicals. Vitamin E may also inhibit blood clot formation and preserve the health of the blood vessels that feed the heart.

The current recommended daily intake of 6 milligrams (9 IU) of vitamin E is based on how much is needed to prevent a deficiency, rather than how much is needed to prevent heart disease. This recommended intake was last revised in 1990. Over the past ten years, our understanding of antioxidant nutrients and disease prevention has rapidly evolved. That's why the National Academy of Science is in the process of establishing new daily recommendations for vitamin E as well as the other dietary antioxidants. At the time of writing this book, the new guidelines had not yet been released. In the meantime, make sure you include food sources of vitamin E in your daily diet. Wheat germ, nuts, seeds, vegetable oils, whole grains, and kale are all good sources. These foods contain vitamin E along with alpha-linolenic acid, an essential fatty acid that I told you earlier might help reduce your risk of heart disease.

But even if you boost your daily intake of vitamin E rich foods, you still won't come close to getting 100 IU, the amount deemed to offer protection in the study of nurses mentioned above. For this reason, you must rely on a supplement. To help you choose the right vitamin E supplement, consider the following suggestions:

- Start by taking 400 IU per day. If you're healthy, there's not much evidence that supports taking more than this. If you have heart disease, some evidence suggests that 800 IU per day is beneficial.
- Buy a "natural source" vitamin E supplement (or look for d-alpha tocopherol on the label; synthetic forms are labeled dl-alpha tocopherol). Although the body absorbs both synthetic and natural vitamin E equally well, your liver prefers the

natural form. It incorporates more natural vitamin E into lipoprotein carrier molecules.

- If you're on blood thinning medication like Coumadin® or Warfarin, don't take vitamin E without consulting your doctor first, as it has slight anti-clotting properties.

LYCOPENE

If you want to add another dietary antioxidant to your dinner plate, consider lycopene. Scientists are only now discovering this compound's role in disease prevention. You might be interested to know that not only is lycopene being studied for its role in heart disease prevention, but also for its potential as an anticancer agent (lycopene may help fight cancers of the prostate, lung, and cervix).

Lycopene is a cousin of beta-carotene, the antioxidant nutrient you eat your carrots for. It turns out that, compared to beta-carotene, lycopene is twice as potent as an antioxidant. Lycopene is found in red coloured fruits and vegetables. It's what gives these foods their bright colour and it also protects these plants from disease. Tomatoes are the richest source of lycopene, but you'll also find some in pink grapefruit, watermelon, guava, and apricots.

Researchers have observed a relationship between the amount of lycopene found in an individual's blood and body fat stores and that individual's risk of developing heart disease. A study looking at participants from ten European countries reported that men with marginal lycopene stores had a 52 percent increased risk of heart attack compared to those individuals with the highest body stores.

As an antioxidant, lycopene provides yet another dietary defense mechanism against free radical damage to LDL cholesterol. Toronto researchers studied the effect of dietary lycopene in 19 healthy adults. A diet supplemented with tomato products doubled lycopene blood levels and significantly reduced free radical damage to LDL cholesterol. Lycopene may also lower the level of LDL cholesterol by hampering its production in the liver. One small study found that a 60-milligram lycopene supplement taken for three months was able to lower LDL levels by 14 percent.[30]

While more work needs to be done to unravel the precise role lycopene plays in heart health, there's no reason to wait for the research to be finished before taking steps to get a good supply in your daily diet—foods containing lycopene are healthy for all sorts of other reasons, anyway. Based on the research that has been conducted, it appears than an intake of five to seven milligrams daily offers protection. And that's easy to get if you eat heat processed tomato products.

LYCOPENE CONTENT OF FOODS (MILLIGRAMS)

Tomato, raw, 1 small	0.8–3.8
Tomatoes, cooked, 1 cup (250 ml)	9.25
Tomato sauce, 1/2 cup (125 ml)	3.1
Tomato paste, 2 tbsp. (25 ml)	8.0
Tomato juice, 1 cup (250 ml)	12.5–29.0
Ketchup, 2 tbsp. (25 ml)	3.1 to 4.2
Apricots, dried, 10 halves	0.3
Grapefruit, pink, 1/2	4.2
Papaya, 1 whole	6.2–16.5
Watermelon, 1 slice, 10 in. (25 cm) x 3/4 in. (2 cm)	8.5–26.4

In addition to the fact that heat processed tomato products give you more lycopenes (as you can easily see in the list above), you'll also be interested to know that it's easier for your body to absorb lycopene from these foods. Even though one fresh tomato packs up to four milligrams of lycopene, your body doesn't absorb all of it. Eat the same tomato from a can, and you'll absorb more of the lycopene it contains. And here's another tip to help you increase the amount of lycopene you absorb—add a little olive oil to your pasta sauce. Lycopene is a fat soluble compound and as a result it's better absorbed in the presence of a little fat.

What about lycopene supplements?

If you're looking for a lycopene boost, all you really have to do is add a glass of low sodium tomato juice to your lunch. However, lycopene supplements are available in health food stores and drug stores. If you opt for a supplement, I recommend that you choose a brand made with either Lyc-O-Mato or LycoRed extract. These extracts come from Israel and are derived from whole tomatoes. They are also the extracts that have been used in clinical studies. Most supplements offer five milligrams of lycopene per tablet, so one a day is all you need.

COENZYME Q10

Here's an antioxidant that you may not have heard about. Coenzyme Q10 (CoQ10) was discovered back in 1957 at the University of Wisconsin. Today, believe it or not, it's one of the top six selling pharmacological agents in Japan. Coenzyme Q10 is also known as ubiquinone (from the word ubiquitous—that's because it is found in all plant and animal cells).

If you haven't heard about CoQ10, it's probably because it is not considered a nutrient—there's no daily recommended intake for this substance. Our cells form CoQ10 with the help of vitamin B6 and amino acid called tyrosine (amino acids are the building blocks of proteins). As we age, our CoQ10 levels decline.

There are two reasons why you should be familiar with this compound. For starters, it is an antioxidant and may prevent free radical damage to LDL cholesterol. In the liver, CoQ10 is packaged into LDL cholesterol molecules, and from there, transported on LDL carriers to other parts of the body. As a part of the LDL particle, CoQ10 is able to neutralize harmful free radicals that attack LDL cholesterol. In fact, CoQ10 levels in your blood may represent the amount of oxidative stress your body is regularly faced with. One study found that, compared to healthy individuals, CoQ10 levels were lower in patients with high cholesterol and in those who smoked. CoQ10 levels were the highest in younger people.

If you're taking medication for high blood cholesterol, you might also consider taking a CoQ10 supplement. That's because the so-called "statin" drugs (such as Mevacor®, Zocor®, Pravachol®, Lescol®, and Lipitor®) have been shown to cause a significant reduction in blood CoQ10 levels. The higher the drug dose taken, the lower CoQ10 levels fall.

If you have heart disease, CoQ10 may help keep your LDL and HDL cholesterol levels within the normal range. Studies from India gave patients 60 milligrams of CoQ10 twice daily and saw not only an improvement of cholesterol levels, but also a reduction in complications during the first 28 days after a heart attack.[31]

Studies have used anywhere from 60 to 120 milligrams of CoQ10 per day. The supplement is well tolerated and no serious side effects have ever been reported with long-term use. Laboratory studies do indicate that supplements containing CoQ10 in an oil base are more available to the body.

herbal remedies

GARLIC

Garlic (*Allium sativum*) contains many different sulfur compounds, and one in particular, called S-allyl cysteine (SAC), appears to lower total cholesterol, LDL cholesterol, and triglycerides, and raise levels of HDL cholesterol. SAC is present in small amounts in raw garlic, but its concentration increases when garlic is aged. The scientific studies that show a positive effect have used an aged garlic extract (Kyolic) to achieve a cholesterol reduction. Aged garlic extract contains many different sulfur compounds but research points to SAC as the compound with the most biological activity.

One American study from Brown University School of Medicine gave 41 men with high cholesterol nine aged garlic capsules (for a total of 7.2 grams) or placebo pills for 6 months. Those taking the garlic tended to show a 7 percent lowering of total cholesterol levels, a 4.6 percent lowering of LDL levels, and a 5.5 percent reduction in blood pressure. Other studies have found 900 milligrams of dried garlic powder in capsule form to be effective at reducing levels of blood cholesterol.[32]

While the findings regarding other forms of garlic have been less consistent, some studies have shown positive results with garlic powder capsules and fresh garlic.

Garlic may reduce the risk of heart disease in a number of ways.

- It inhibits cholesterol production in the liver.
- It lowers blood triglyceride levels.
- It thins the blood and reduces the stickiness of platelets.
- It acts as an antioxidant and prevents damage or oxidation to LDL cholesterol (many studies have found SAC in aged garlic extract to significantly inhibit free radical damage to LDL cholesterol).
- It lowers blood pressure.

When it comes to fresh garlic we don't yet know the optimal intake needed for heart health. Many scientists agree that as little as one-half clove each day will offer health benefits. Most people can take one or two cloves a day (about 3 to 6 grams raw garlic) without any problems. Some people, however, are sensitive to garlic. The oil soluble compounds in fresh garlic account for its potential to upset the stomach and to cause that wonderful smell.

I encourage you to use more garlic in cooking. Add it to sauces, soups, casseroles, and raw to salad dressings. By using raw, cooked, and, if you choose, an aged garlic supplement, you get a variety of protective sulfur compounds. You should also know that although raw garlic contains very little SAC, a recent study from Penn State University found that if you let crushed garlic sit at room temperature for 10 minutes before cooking with it, more beneficial allyl sulfur compounds will be formed.

What about a supplement?

When it comes to garlic supplements, the scientific research points to aged garlic extract as the supplement of choice because of its higher concentration of SAC. Generally, experts recommend taking from one to nine capsules daily (take one to three at a time, with a meal). Because garlic can thin the blood, it should not be used if you are taking blood thinning medications like Coumadin® or Warfarin. If you're taking an aspirin a day, make sure you inform your physician that you have started on garlic.

GUGGUL

Although not technically an herbal remedy, this plant-based product has a long tradition of use in Ayurvedic medicine, the traditional medicine of India. Only recently has it made its way to the western world. Today you'll find supplements of guggul, or guggulipid, in health food stores. These products are made of myrrh, a resin that comes from the bark of the *Commiphora mukul* plant.

Guggul's claim to fame is its cholesterol and triglyceride lowering ability. Studies conducted in India have demonstrated that guggul can significantly lower these blood fats. One study measured the effect of adding 50 milligrams of guggulipid twice daily to a low fat, high fibre diet in 61 patients with high cholesterol levels. All participants followed a cholesterol lowering diet for 12 weeks during which time LDL cholesterol and triglycerides fell. For the next 12 weeks, participants continued their diet but half of them were given guggul and the remaining participants were given a placebo capsule. At the end of the study, those taking guggul were doing significantly better than the participants on placebo. The addition of the resin reduced both LDL cholesterol and triglycerides another 12 percent.[33]

If you have high blood cholesterol and you want to add guggal to your cholesterol lowering regime, you should be aware that it has not been well studied. We know very little about its safety or long term efficacy (in fact, I had difficulty finding much information at all about the product). For this reason, many herbalists don't recommend its use. I have only included it in my book because it is becoming widely available in health food stores. In fact, recently I've had a number of clients ask me about the product. If you do decide to give guggual a try, you should buy a product that states the amount of guggulsterone on the label. According to some experts, 25 milligrams of guggulsterone taken three times daily is the effective dose.

THE bottom LINE...

Leslie's recommendations for reducing your risk of heart disease

1   To keep your cholesterol levels in the healthy range, reduce your intake of saturated fat. Remember to buy low fat milk products: skim or 1% milkfat (MF) milk, yogurt with 1.5% MF or less, and cheese with less than 20% MF. Choose lean cuts of meat and poultry such as inside round, flank steak, sirloin, pork tenderloin and chicken or turkey breast. And use butter sparingly.

2   To eat less trans fat, avoid as much as possible foods that contain partially hydrogenated vegetable oils. If you use margarine, choose one labeled "non-hydrogenated" or make sure that grams of polyunsaturated and monounsaturated fats add up to 6 grams or more per two teaspoon serving.

3   Be sure to include the heart healthy omega-3 fats (a type of polyunsaturated fat) in your diet. Aim to eat fish three times a week.

4   To increase your intake of alpha-linolenic acid, a member of the omega-3 family, use flaxseed oil, walnut oil, and/or canola oil. You can also include a 1/4 cup (50 millilitre) serving of nuts in your diet up to five times a week.

5   If you use olive oil, buy the extra virgin type. It's been processed the least and contains the most antioxidant compounds.

6   If your cholesterol levels are in the normal range, feel free to eat an egg up to six times a week.

7   If your cholesterol levels are high, add 25 grams of soy protein to your diet each day.

8   Every day, include a source of soluble fibre in your diet. Foods like psyllium-enriched breakfast cereals, oatmeal, and oat bran do lower elevated cholesterol in conjunction with a low fat diet, and they also help sustain your energy levels for a longer period of time.

9   When it comes to buying breads, cereals, rice, and pasta always choose whole grain products.

10 Drink a cup (or more) of tea as part of your daily diet to get a source of catechins, antioxidant compounds that protect LDL cholesterol.

11 If you drink alcohol, limit your intake to no more than one alcoholic beverage per day.

12 Boost your intake of B vitamins to help keep your homocysteine levels down. Food sources of B12, B6, and folate can be found on pages 25, 35, and 216. To ensure you are meeting your needs, take a daily multivitamin and mineral supplement or try a B-complex supplement.

13 Eat at least one food rich in vitamin C each day. As an important dietary antioxidant, vitamin C protects your LDL cholesterol from damage caused by free radical molecules. If you're concerned that you are not getting enough vitamin C every day, add 500 or 600 milligrams of Ester-C® to your supplement regime.

14 For even more antioxidant protection, add vitamin E to your daily diet. Wheat germ, nuts and seeds, and kale are good sources. To get the amount of vitamin E found protective in the research, take a daily vitamin E supplement (400 or 800 IU).

15 Each day include a source of lycopene, a cousin of beta-carotene. Just like vitamins C and E, lycopene is an antioxidant and may even help to lower high blood cholesterol. Heat processed tomato products are the best food sources, but look on page 176 for more. If you want to take a lycopene supplement, buy a brand that contains the Lyc-O-Mato or LycoRed extract.

16 If you're currently taking "statin" drugs to lower your cholesterol, take 60 to 120 milligrams of coenzyme Q10 (CoQ10) daily. These drugs lower your body's CoQ10 levels, and CoQ10 is yet another important antioxidant. You'll find a list of these drugs on page 177.

17 To get more heart protective sulfur compounds, increase your intake of garlic, both raw and cooked. Use one-half to one clove each day in cooking. If your cholesterol levels are high, consider taking aged garlic extract (it's odourless too!). Take one to two capsules (300 to 600 milligrams) up to three times daily with meals. If you are on blood thinning medication, be sure to check with your physician or pharmacist for possible side effects or interactions.

18 If you have a high cholesterol level and you're wondering about guggul, or guggulipid, be wary. Few studies have been done to assess this product's safety or long-term efficacy. Based on what is known, the effective dose may be 25 milligrams of guggulsterone three times daily.

reducing your risk of breast cancer

"There are only two types of women today: women who have breast cancer and women who are afraid they are going to get breast cancer."

10

The thought of breast cancer probably scares women more than the spectre of any other type of cancer. With menopause the fear often becomes magnified—most of us know that the risk of developing cancer increases with age, and we are also concerned about hormone replacement therapy and its possible effect on our breasts. As with any other disease, some things encourage cancer and other things discourage it, and our knowledge of factors influencing cancer in general, and breast cancer in particular, is growing steadily. I hope that after you read this chapter you will feel ready to take a proactive approach to reducing your cancer risk. As you will see, there is plenty of action you can take.

statistics on breast cancer

Breast cancer is the most common type of cancer among Canadian women. The Canadian Cancer Society estimated that 18,700 new cases of breast cancer would develop in 1999, representing 30 percent of all cancers (official figures won't be released until later in the year 2000). Breast cancer deaths in 1999 were estimated at 5,400, accounting for 18 percent of all cancer deaths (lung cancer tops the list, followed by breast, then colon cancer). Sadly, fifteen Canadian women die every day from breast cancer. But the good news is that the death rate from breast cancer has decreased by 10 percent since 1986. This is largely due to the fact that more and more women are having mammograms, allowing for earlier detection (more on mammograms later in this chapter).

Most women want to know what their risk of developing this disease is, and what they can do to prevent it. The following table shows you the risk of developing breast cancer by a certain age.

LIFETIME BREAST CANCER RISK

Age	Risk
25 years	less than 1 in 1,000
50 years	1 in 63
75 years	1 in 15
90 years	1 in 9

These numbers mean that by the age of 50, 1 in every 63 women (1.5 percent) will get breast cancer. By the age of 90, 1 in every 9 women will get the disease (11 percent). As you read these numbers, keep in mind that statistical risks can't be applied to you as an individual. They represent the average risk for the entire population of Canadian women. If you have certain risk factors for breast cancer, such as a family history of breast cancer or a poor diet, these numbers underestimate your risk. Conversely, if you have no risk factors at all for the disease, the numbers above will overestimate your chances of getting breast cancer.

At this point, you're probably wondering what factors can increase your odds of getting breast cancer. But before we get to that, I want take you through a short pathology (the study of diseases) course. If you understand the cancer process, it might help to ease your worry that cancer is an inevitable disease.

cancer

Simply put, cancer is a disease in which abnormal cells grow out of control. When enough of these cells accumulate, a tumor forms. If the cancer cells are able to break away from the tumor, they can circulate throughout the body and take up residence in another organ, a process called metastasis. But let's go back to the earliest steps in cancer development.

Cancer begins at the cellular level. Normally our body cells divide every day in order to repair damaged tissues, replace old cells, and grow new tissue. Normal cell growth and division is regulated by internal controls. For instance, if you cut yourself, your body will release messenger chemicals to tell cells in the wounded area to quickly divide and make new cells. Certain receptors on your cells receive the messenger chemicals and then trigger specific enzymes to speed up cellular division. When your wound has healed, the delivery of these messenger chemicals is shut off and cellular life returns to normal. Besides the types of controls that take care of healing, healthy cells are also programmed to die at a certain age so that cellular death will be in balance with new cell growth. But sometimes the process can go awry. Cells don't stop dividing even though your body tells them to. They take on a life of their own and grow in an unregulated fashion. These cells don't die when they are programmed to. This is what happens in cancer.

WHAT MAKES A CELL CANCEROUS?

Every cell has a genetic blueprint, called deoxyribonucleic acid (DNA). The DNA of cells contains genes that program cell reproduction, growth, and repair of all body tissues. Sometimes genes can become damaged and this damage can result in cancer. In essence, there are three ways in which your genes can become faulty:

- A mutation can occur during normal cell division such that the newly formed cell contains an abnormal gene. This can happen randomly or if the cell is exposed to some other agent.
- Cells might be exposed to an environmental agent, called a carcinogen, that harms the DNA. For instance, cigarette smoking is a carcinogen that promotes the development of lung cancer.
- Flawed genes can be inherited from your parents. Very few cancers are actually the result of inherited genes.

Just because you have one damaged gene does not mean you are destined to get cancer. Many processes must take place before a cancer develops. Your body has what are called tumor suppressor genes which keep an eye out for damaged DNA and halt it in its tracks. But if these tumor suppressor genes become mutated, then cells with abnormal genes can multiply at an uncontrolled rate. It is estimated that in 20 to 40 percent of breast cancer cases a particular tumor suppressor gene (called p53) is mutated. Several genetic mutations are probably needed for breast cancer to develop. Genes that go on to cause cancer are called oncogenes.

Cancer is not explained by genetics alone. For instance, some people who have a family history of a certain cancer never end up getting that cancer. Experts agree that cancer is the result of an *interaction* between genes and environmental factors, like diet. For instance, you might have a mutated gene that predisposes you to breast cancer, but because you eat a low fat diet high in antioxidant-rich fruits and vegetables, you may never get cancer. On the other hand, if you are regularly exposed to pollutants and eat a poor diet, the risk that any faulty genes you carry will catalyze a cancerous growth is increased.

how breast cancer develops

The breast is comprised mainly of fatty tissue which gives it its size and shape. Within this fatty tissue are milk glands. Lobules are groups of individual milk-forming glands and each lobule empties into a duct, a small passageway that carries milk to the nipple. It's in the lobules and ducts that most breast cancer begins. Within the breast is also a network of lymphatic vessels, which connect to lymph nodes under the arm, under the collarbone, and near the breastbone. The lymphatic system drains fluid and particles (called lymph) from the breast into the lymph nodes. The lymph then enters the bloodstream and is eventually removed from the body.

Breast cancer begins with a single cell that runs amok, usually in the lobule or duct. Cancers probably start here because these are two areas where cells divide rapidly during the normal menstrual cycle. Estrogen and progesterone stimulate the breast cells to begin dividing each month, preparing the body for pregnancy. If conception does not occur, breast cell receptors receive a message to stop cell division. The process begins again the following month, and every month in which menstruation occurs, until menopause. Because fairly rapid cell division occurs regularly in the breast for such a span of years, there is a greater chance for a genetic mutation to occur. While most breast cancers are not detected until after menopause, it is believed that the majority actually begin to develop in the premenopausal years.

BREAST CANCER GENES

Some cases of breast cancer are caused by inherited mutations in the genes BRCA1 and BRCA2. The gene BRCA1 was identified in 1994 and in its mutated form is now believed to cause inherited early-onset breast cancer; this disease accounts for five percent of breast cancers. BRCA1 is actually a tumor suppressor gene, the type of gene that's supposed to work to keep DNA healthy. Families carrying a faulty BRCA1 gene experience a high incidence of both breast and ovarian cancers that occur at a young age. However, 80 percent of breast cancers occur in older women who don't have the flawed BRCA1 gene. Genetic testing that screens for faulty BRCA1 and BRCA2 genes is available across Canada. Testing is done at what are usually called Familial Breast Cancer Clinics, often connected to a cancer treatment centre. Eligibility for the test will vary depending on the province in which you live. Usually you will be eligible if you have two or more close relatives with breast cancer and a referral from your physician. At the clinic, a woman will be counselled as to the pros and cons of having such a test. If she decides to take it, she will be counselled as to how to deal with the ramifications of the results.

Genetic tests, I am sure, will add a great deal of worry to many women's lives. It will become important to remember that not all mutated genes go on to catalyze a cancer. And in the case of those who find they have the mutated BRCA1 or BRCA2 gene, this information will no doubt be used to spur important preventative decisions in response to a higher breast cancer risk.

RISK FACTORS FOR BREAST CANCER

While we don't yet know all the causes of breast cancer, ongoing research is adding to our knowledge base at a rapid speed. Studies of large numbers of women have been able to identify risk factors that increase a woman's chance of developing breast cancer. To date, the clearest risk factors for the disease are associated with hormonal and reproductive factors. Exactly how hormones play a role is not yet fully understood. However, researchers do believe that estrogen can promote the growth and development of mutated breast cells. As you will see below, a common thread in many of the identified risk factors is the length of time your breast tissue has been exposed to your body's circulating estrogen via the menstrual cycle. The longer the exposure, the greater the risk of breast cancer.

Age

As you saw in the risk chart above, breast cancer is more common in women over 50 years of age. In fact, more than 75 percent of breast cancers occur in post-menopausal women. While it is possible to develop breast cancer at a younger age, most women don't. Keep in mind also that increasing age makes other risk factors discussed below more likely to occur. When two or more risk factors are combined, your risk becomes greater than when you have been exposed to one risk factor alone.

Previous breast cancer

A history of breast cancer increases the odds that a woman will get breast cancer again, in both the same and the opposite breast.

Family history

If you have a first degree relative with breast cancer (a mother or a sister) your risk of developing the disease is approximately doubled, and you run an even greater risk if more than one close relative is affected, or if the cancer has occurred at a young age in a first degree family member. But while it is true that breast cancer in the family increases risk, the additional risk may not be as great as you think. If you have a breast cancer gene there is a 50 percent chance you will pass it on to your daughter. If she, in turn, gets the gene, there is a 50 percent chance that she will pass it on to her child, and so on. Purely hereditary breast cancer accounts for only 5 to 10 percent of all cases. And remember, even if you are unlucky enough to inherit a breast cancer causing gene, you are not fated to get the disease. You can take preventive action.

Age at first pregnancy

Women who have children before 30 years of age have a lower risk of developing breast cancer. Women who have their first child after 30 have a higher risk and women who never have children are at an even greater risk. Many experts believe that the important factor here is the amount of time that lapses between menarche (the onset of menstruation) and first pregnancy. The theory is that the developing breast tissue is most sensitive to cancer causing agents (carcinogens) during this time. Hormones produced only during pregnancy mature the breast cells and make them more resistant to carcinogens. It may be that these same pregnancy hormones stimulate mutated breast cells in a woman who has her first baby after 30 years of age.

Age at first period

If your period began before you were 12 years of age, you have, statistically speaking, a slightly higher risk of developing breast cancer. In fact, each year that puberty is delayed may offer as much as a 20 percent reduction in risk. Many of the changes that occur at puberty are due to higher levels of endogenous estrogen (estrogen that's made in your body). It is believed that the longer breast tissue is exposed to higher levels of endogenous estrogen, the greater the chance for cells to become cancerous.

Late menopause

Women who menstruate for longer than 40 years have a slightly higher risk of breast cancer. Like early menarche, late menopause influences the amount of time breast cells are exposed to estrogen.

The list above describes the stronger risk factors for the disease. In addition, however, the following factors may play a role, but they are less well understood:

Exposure to radiation

Radiation from X-rays taken during a woman's younger years may increase the risk for breast cancer later in life. It appears that this factor is more significant if exposure occurs before the age of 40. Despite this fact, experts feel exposure to radiation is probably a minor contribution to overall risk.

Use of hormones

In animal studies, estrogen intake is associated with an increased occurrence of breast cancer. In women, however, the effects of supplemental hormones are less clear. Studies have failed to show an increased risk of breast cancer in younger women who take birth control pills. When it comes to hormone replacement therapy, short-term use is considered safe. But there is a concern if hormones are taken for more than 10 years, or if women with a family history of breast cancer take them. In these cases HRT may increase the risk slightly, but more research is needed. One recent large study found that taking HRT for more than 5 years increased the risk of breast cancer by 2.6 times (260 percent) in the 37,000 women studied.[1] Clearly the pros and cons of HRT need to be discussed with your physician.

Diet

More and more studies are determining that certain dietary factors increase the risk of developing breast cancer. Diet affects breast cancer development by either initiating cancer growth through causing a genetic mutation, or by promoting the growth of cancerous cells. This chapter includes an extensive discussion of the many dietary and nutritional factors that have been studied in relation to breast cancer risk.

SCREENING FOR BREAST CANCER

The larger and more well established a breast cancer tumor is, the more difficult it is to treat. This is especially true if the tumor metastasizes before treatment begins. Experts agree that your best protection against breast cancer is prevention, and that's what I'll discuss in most of the rest of this chapter. If you do develop a tumor, the earliest possible detection makes successful treatment more likely. For that reason, it's also important to use the methods currently available for early detection.

Mammograms

Around the time of menopause is when you should be thinking about getting your first mammogram. Doctors recommend that all Canadian women between the ages of 50 and 69 have a mammogram every two years in combination with a physical exam of the breasts by a trained health professional. A mammogram is a special X-ray of the breast that will reveal the location of a breast lump, its size, and certain characteristics that may be suggestive of cancer. If a lump looks suspicious to your physician, further tests will be done to determine if it's malignant. Mammograms use very low doses of radiation and do not cause breast cancer; nor do they make an existing cancer worse. Rather, a mammogram is a very important screening tool that can catch breast cancer early.

Not all lumps are seen on a mammogram. Younger women have denser breasts, which make detection more difficult. This is one of the reasons why women under 50 are not encouraged to have regular mammograms (also because breast cancer is less common in premenopausal women).

While it is generally accepted that mammograms save the lives of women who are over 50 years of age, there is debate on whether women in the premenopausal transitional years between 40 and 49 should start having routine mammograms. Currently, because of the results of the Canadian National Breast Screening Study, health authorities do not recommend routine mammograms for this age group. In this 10-year study of 25,000 40- to 49-year-old women, there was no difference in breast cancer death rates between women who were screened and women who were not.[2]

Breast self-exam

Although less reliable at detecting cancer than a mammogram combined with a physical examination by your doctor, the breast self-exam is an important way to detect physical changes in your breasts. By the age of 40, all Canadian women should be performing monthly breast self-exams. Use the pads of your fingers to examine the tissue in your breasts and in your armpits. Breast self-exams should be done at the same point during each menstrual cycle. Be sure to also look carefully at your breasts in the mirror. Any of the following changes, whether detected manually or visually, should prompt a visit to your family doctor:

- A lump or thick area in the breast or underarm area.
- Unusual swelling of the breast.
- Change in colour or texture of the skin on the breast.
- Blood leakage from the nipple or areola (the dark ring surrounding the nipple).
- Inversion of the nipple (the nipple puckers inwards, rather than pointing outwards).

PREVENTING BREAST CANCER

Changing your lifestyle

Factors such as lifestyle and diet definitely make a difference to your risk of developing many types of cancer. In 1997, an international expert panel of the World Cancer Research Fund and the American Institute for Cancer Research released a 653-page report that outlined dietary advice to prevent cancer. The report stated that between 30 and 40 percent of all cancer cases are preventable by a healthy diet, regular exercise, and maintaining a healthy weight. The report went on to say that diets high in fruits and vegetables could alone prevent at least 20 percent of all cancer cases.[3]

When it comes to breast cancer, dietary factors such as fat, alcohol, fibre, and fruits and vegetables have all been well studied. Below are my nutrition recommendations based on our current scientific knowledge. While some of these strategies have strong research to support their adoption, others do not have such strong evidence backing them. However, evidence does exist to suggest that they *may* be helpful. And certainly when it comes to eating a low fat diet packed with fibre and antioxidant nutrients, I really don't think you can go wrong. While we are still learning about breast cancer, making the dietary changes I list below will help you improve your overall well-being. And they just might lower your odds of getting breast cancer.

dietary strategies

DIETARY FAT

When most women think of diet and breast cancer they think of fat. The main hypothesis among nutrition researchers has long been that a high fat diet increases the risk of getting the disease. And certainly no other nutrient has been studied so heavily with respect to breast cancer. Throughout the 1980s and 1990s, however, the fat hypothesis has come under debate. It seems the high fat diet/breast cancer link is not as clear-cut as we had thought.

Scientists became interested in the link between fat intake and breast cancer when they noticed that women in countries with low fat intakes had much lower rates of breast cancer as compared to women in countries with higher fat diets. It has been hypothesized that dietary fat may increase breast cancer risk by increasing estrogen production (you'll recall I told you earlier that a woman's circulating estrogen is thought to be related to breast cancer risk by stimulating the growth of breast tissue). Studies do show that vegetarian women who have low fat, high fibre diets have lower levels of estrogen and less breast cancer.[4] Another way high fat diets may cause breast cancer is through weight gain and body fat accumulation, which in turn increases the risk of breast cancer. That's because fat cells produce estrogen.

Theory aside, does the amount of fat you eat make a difference to your risk? In animal studies, very high fat diets stimulate breast cancer growth, but this effect has not been seen in human studies. Most large studies have failed to show a strong relationship between total fat intake and breast cancer risk. Toronto researchers summarized 23 studies done up until 1993 and concluded that a high fat diet increased the risk of breast cancer by about 12 percent. A recent 14-year study of 89,000 women found no evidence that a high fat diet promoted breast cancer or that a low fat diet protected against it. Many experts, however, believe that the women in these studies didn't reduce their fat intake enough to see a benefit.[5] Health Canada's recommendation of "no more that 30 percent of your daily calories from fat" might be too high to offer protection from breast cancer.

A large Toronto study is currently underway to determine if a very low fat diet can prevent breast cancer. So far the results look promising. One report found that women who ate a low fat (21 percent), high carbohydrate (61 percent) diet for two years had significantly reduced dense breast areas as seen by mammogram (dense breast areas are a risk factor for cancer), as compared to women on a 30 percent fat diet. Another report from this research group revealed that women who followed a 15 percent fat diet for two years had lower levels of circulating estrogen, which could offer protection.[6] We won't know whether these two findings will translate into a lower rate of breast cancer in the women in these studies consuming a low fat diet until a longer period of time has passed. But based on these initial reports, I certainly believe that following a low fat diet is a wise precautionary measure.

In addition to studying how much fat a woman eats, researchers have been busy looking at the different types of fat and their effects on breast cancer. Before we look at what they've found, it's important that you understand the differences between the various fats found in food.

Saturated fat

Chemically speaking, when fat is saturated, it will be hard at room temperature. Animal fat is saturated—a block of butter or the marbled fat in meat and poultry are examples of fats that are solid at room temperature. The fat in cheese, milk, and eggs is also saturated. Finally, certain vegetable oils can be saturated too. These are oils that have been hydrogenated to make them hard and increase their shelf life. Manufacturers add hydrogenated vegetable oils to commercial products. These oils add crunch to store-bought cookies and snack foods, and make them last longer.

Polyunsaturated fat

This term refers to fats that are liquid at room temperature. Think of a bottle of vegetable oil, be it corn, sunflower, safflower, or sesame. These oils are all polyunsaturated fats and belong to the omega-6 family. Special types of fat called omega-3 fats are found in fish and are also polyunsaturated. The oilier the fish, the more polyunsaturated fat it contains. Omega-3 fats are also found in flaxseed oil and walnut oil.

Monounsaturated fat

This fat is a little different from the two described above. If you refrigerate a monounsaturated fat, it turns semi-solid. If you take it out of the fridge and store it at room temperature it will return to a liquid form. Chances are you're already familiar with monounsaturated fats—olive oil, canola oil, and peanut oil are your best sources. (And if you're wondering why canola oil doesn't get as hard as olive oil when you refrigerate it, it's because canola actually contains both monounsaturated and polyunsaturated fat.)

Saturated fat, meat, and milk

Several studies have looked at the relationship between foods high in saturated fat—meat and dairy products—and breast cancer. When it comes to meat, the findings are mixed. Some studies show that higher meat intakes are linked with a greater risk, whereas others don't show any effect. Based on a review of the research, the international panel of experts from the World Cancer Research Fund and the American Institute for Cancer Research, mentioned above, recently concluded that meat might possibly increase a woman's risk.

The harmful effect of meat may be due to its saturated fat content, or it may be due to the way it's prepared. Cooking meat at high temperatures forms compounds called *heterocyclic amines* which have been shown to cause breast tumors in animals. It appears that well-done meat may not be that healthy for women either. Researchers at the University of Minnesota have learned that women who eat their hamburger, steak, and bacon well done are more than four times as likely to have breast cancer than women who enjoy their meat rare or medium done.[7] Until we know more about the effects of cooked meat, breast cancer experts advise that we consume no more than 3 ounces (90 grams) of meat each day.

As for dairy products, not all the studies looking at the relationship between dairy products and breast cancer have reported a higher risk from dairy consumption. In fact, a recent Finnish study suggests that drinking a glass of whole milk might offer protection against breast cancer. Researchers in Helsinki studied 4,697 women for 25 years and discovered that those participants who had the highest intake of milk had a 48 percent lower risk of developing breast cancer than the women who drank the least.

Scientists speculate that a special fat might be responsible for milk's protective effect. Conjugated linoleic acid (CLA) occurs naturally in milk (and meat) and has been shown in a number of animal studies to inhibit breast cancer growth.[8] Scientists believe that CLA protects cells from becoming cancerous when breast cells are dividing.

Polyunsaturated fat and fish

In animals, very high intakes of polyunsaturated vegetable oils can promote breast tumor growth. But keep in mind that the studies that came to these conclusions were looking at animals fed 45 percent of their calories from fat. That's pretty high. The average Canadian eats less fat than that, getting more like 32 percent of daily calories in the form of fat. The data on humans shows that vegetable oils have no effect on breast cancer risk, at least in the amounts we typically consume. So there's no need to throw away your bottle of sunflower seed oil!

You may want to start eating more fish. In studied populations, women who eat plenty of fish for many years have a lower incidence of breast cancer. And while no trials have been done in women, one experimental study did find that omega-3 fats from fish oil actually suppressed human breast cancer cell growth and metastatic cancer in female mice (scientists inject human breast cancer cells into mice to study the effects of different carcinogens).[9] Although there is not a lot of evidence for fish's protective effect, the existing studies do suggest that you get more omega-3 fats into your diet. My recommendation is to eat fish three times a week. Before you say "no way," take a look at a few of my tasty ways to cook your fish, on page 196. If you try these recipes you just might think twice. Actually, there was a time not too long ago when my husband wouldn't go near anything with fins. Today we eat fish more often than chicken and meat combined.

NUTRITION TIP

Three tasty ways to serve (and enjoy!) fish

Looking for ways to sneak fish onto your family's dinner plate—or your own? Try these quick ideas that pack flavour and omega-3s—no measuring necessary!

Lemon dilled salmon

Place a salmon filet or salmon steak on a piece of aluminum foil. Squeeze the juice of 1/2 lemon over the fish and top with fresh chopped dill and black pepper. Wrap up in foil and bake at 400 degrees Fahrenheit (205 degrees Celsius) for 25 minutes.

Hoisin salmon

Mix hoisin sauce with a touch of hot chili paste chopped fresh ginger, and a little roasted sesame oil. Brush over fish. Bake at 425 degrees Fahrenheit (220 degrees Celsius) for 12 to 14 minutes or until done to your liking.

Asian-style marinated fish

Marinate a filet or steak of white fish (halibut, swordfish, sea bass) in a ziploc bag for 30 minutes with Mo's Authentic Japanese dressing. (Mo's is my favourite brand, but you can use any product you like.) If you don't have time to marinate the fish, drizzle about 1/4 cup (50 ml) of the dressing over the fish just before baking. Bake at 425 degrees Fahrenheit (220 degrees Celsius) for 12 to 14 minutes or until done to your liking. For a different flavour, try using oyster sauce.

Monounsaturated fat and olive oil

No doubt you've read that olive oil is good for your heart. But can it help you reduce your odds of developing breast cancer too? It's true that breast cancer is less common in Mediterranean countries where olive oil is the main source of fat. A few studies have even found that women with breast cancer use significantly less olive oil compared to women free of the disease.[10] I've already told you that olive oil is a rich source of monounsaturated fat. Could this be the protective factor? Or perhaps the secret ingredients are olive oil's natural antioxidants, like vitamin E? Researchers don't think so. At this time there appears to be no relationship between monounsaturated fat or vitamin E and breast cancer risk. It may be that if you consume more olive oil, you eat less of other fats that might increase your risk (like saturated fat).

SOY FOODS

We're back to soy again. You can't escape the health benefits of this humble bean. Populations (including Japanese people and vegetarians) who consume the largest amounts of soy have the lowest rates of breast cancer. Researchers attribute soy's possible protective effect to naturally occurring compounds called isoflavones. When we consume soy foods, bacteria in our intestinal tract convert isoflavones to compounds that act like a weak estrogen hormone in the body. That's why isoflavones are called phytoestrogens (plant estrogens). Two soy isoflavones called genistein and diadzein have been studied extensively.

Acting as weak estrogen compounds, isoflavones are able to attach to estrogen receptors in the body. In fact, genistein has a much stronger pull to certain estrogen receptors than does estradiol, one of your body's own estrogen hormones. Researchers believe that if genistein can bind to estrogen receptors in the breast, it blocks a woman's own estrogen from taking those spots. And that's good news because it means that breast cells have less contact with estrogen.

A regular intake of soy isoflavones may also alter hormone production and lower levels of circulating hormones in the bloodstream. A small study done at the University of Texas found that premenopausal women who drank three 12-ounce (375-millilitre) glasses of soy beverage each day had lower blood levels of estrogen than women on a soy-free diet. The lower estrogen levels lasted up to three menstrual cycles after the women stopped taking the soy. A Tufts University study presented at the 1999 Third International Symposium on the Role of Soy in Preventing and Treating Chronic Disease in Washington, DC also found that a high soy diet lowered blood estrogen by 20 percent in menopausal women.

A high soy diet can also influence how much estrogen your breast cells come in contact with by lengthening the menstrual cycle slightly. One study showed that a daily intake of soy products containing 45 milligrams of isoflavones lengthened the menstrual cycle of premenopausal women.[11] Over a lifetime, longer menstrual cycles mean fewer menstrual cycles; this, in turn, means the breasts receive less exposure to estrogen.

Whether the ability of soy isoflavones to influence hormone levels in our body can prevent breast cancer remains to be seen. No study has been done yet to show what years of eating a high soy diet does to breast cancer risk. I can tell you that most experts who are studying soy isoflavones agree that you probably have to start eating soy foods at a very young age to get protection from breast cancer.

If you're a breast cancer survivor you might be leery about eating foods containing plant estrogens. If isoflavones can bind to breast estrogen receptors, can they stimulate the growth of breast tissue as estrogen does? Studies have found that a diet rich in soy isoflavones actually *reduces* the growth of breast tumors in mice. Laboratory research has also found that genistein inhibits the growth of estrogen-positive and estrogen-negative human breast cancer cells.[12] (In case you're wondering about these terms, let me explain briefly. Postmenopausal women tend to get estrogen-positive tumors. The cells in an estrogen-positive tumor have estrogen receptors and will respond to estrogen. In general, these tumors have a better prognosis than estrogen-negative tumours because they are slower growing and they respond to hormone treatments. Premenopausal women are more likely to get an estrogen-negative tumor, which rarely responds to hormonal treatments since the cells in it do not have estrogen receptors.)

While these studies show that soy has an anti-estrogen effect and prevents breast cancer cells from growing, a few laboratory studies suggest that high intakes of genistein might enhance breast tissue growth. British researchers studied the effect of a 60-gram soy supplement (containing 45 milligrams isoflavones) in 48 premenopausal women with benign breast disease or breast cancer. Soy supplementation for two weeks did stimulate growth of normal breast cells.[13] This finding does not mean, however, that short term soy consumption increases the chance of breast cancer. Rather, it means we need more research in this area to understand how soy works in women with breast cancer.

To date, most evidence suggests that a long-term intake of soy foods prevents breast cancer from developing in the first place. Unfortunately, there are no specific recommendations for women with estrogen-positive breast cancer because the research has not been done. For women with estrogen positive breast cancer, the decision to use soy products is a personal one. Until we know more and I can confidently give women with previous breast cancer advice, I recommend that you stick to eating natural soy foods (like soybeans, tofu, soy beverages) and avoid supplements that contain concentrated amounts of isoflavones.

If you want to start eating soy foods because they *might* help reduce your risk of breast cancer *and* because they have many other health benefits (if you haven't already, read Chapter 9 on soy's cholesterol lowering power), try adding one soy food to your diet each day. Chapter 1 outlines different types of soy foods and how to enjoy them.

FLAXSEED

The tiny brown or golden seeds known as flax are now being studied for their possible role in preventing breast cancer. Flaxseed contains natural compounds, called lignans (you might also be interested to know that flax seeds are rich in soluble fibre and an essential fatty acid called alpha-linolenic acid). When we eat flaxseed, bacteria in our gut convert the plant lignans into human lignans, which act very much like estrogen in the body. Once in the body, phytoestrogens from flaxseed have a weak estrogen-like action and are able to bind to estrogen receptors. In so doing, they can, like other phytoestrogens, help block the action of our body's own potent estrogen on breast cells.

Two studies conducted at the University of Toronto found that lignans from flaxseed reduced the size of breast tumors in rats.[14] Whether flaxseed can do this in humans is another question. And it's a question that's being addressed now by Dr. Lillian Anderson and her team at the University of Toronto. In their study, women with breast cancer are being given 25 grams of flaxseed daily, in the form of a muffin, to see if the flaxseed lignans have any beneficial effect on tumor size between diagnosis and surgery. Unfortunately, at the time of writing, study results are not yet in. But stay tuned.

In the meantime, should you be eating flax? It's too early to say that eating flaxseed will reduce breast cancer risk, but you can still make it part of your regular diet, just in case. It certainly won't do you any harm. If nothing else, you'll add a source of fibre and essential fat to your diet. Aim to get one to two tablespoons (15 to 25 millilitres) of ground flaxseed each day. It is very important that you grind your flaxseed in order to release the lignans. Otherwise all you'll be getting is a source of fibre. Grind flaxseed in a clean coffee grinder or use a mortle and pestle. You can also buy it pre-ground at health food stores but it is more expensive (Omega Nutrition makes a good product).

Now the real question: what do you do with it? Plenty! Here are just a few ideas that will add crunch and a great nutty flavour to your meals:

- Add ground flaxseed to hot cereals, pancakes, muffin batters, and cookie mixes. I have clients who even add it to cold breakfast cereal!
- Mix ground flaxseed into yogurt.
- Sprinkle flax on salads and soups.
- Add flaxseed to casseroles.

- Try a loaf of flaxseed bread. Check your local bakery, health food store, or supermarket.
- Try Red River cereal, another good source of flaxseed.

Once you grind flaxseed, be sure to store it (along with your whole seeds) in an airtight container in the fridge or freezer. The natural fats in flaxseed go rancid quickly if exposed to air and heat.

What about flax oil?

I've had many clients tell me they add flaxseed oil to their foods or take flaxseed oil capsules with their morning juice. When I ask them why, many reply "to protect myself from breast cancer." I then explain to them what I'm about to tell you. Flaxseed oil is a great source of alpha-linolenic acid (ALA), an essential fatty acid that our body needs to get from food (ALA belongs to the omega-3 family). But it is not a good source of lignans—the phytoestrogens that may protect the breast. Lignans are found in the seed, along with ALA and fibre. So if you're looking to add to your arsenal of breast cancer fighting foods, your best choice is ground flaxseed, not flax oil.

FRUITS AND VEGETABLES

Looks like Mom was right when she told you to finish your vegetables. Over 200 studies from around the world have shown that a diet high in fruits and vegetables lowers the risk of developing many cancers, including breast cancer. American researchers from Harvard University studied more than 89,000 women and found that those who ate more than 2.2 servings of vegetables daily had a 20 percent lower risk of breast cancer than those who ate less than one serving. Another study of premenopausal women found that high total vegetable intake lowered the risk of breast cancer by 54 percent.[15]

It appears that dark green vegetables, which contain beta-carotene, other carotenoid compounds, and folate (a B vitamin) are most protective. Beta-carotene is an antioxidant nutrient, which means it is able to protect cells from damage caused by harmful free radical molecules. Our bodies form free radicals from oxygen every day as a consequence of normal metabolism. Pollution and cigarette smoke increase free radical levels in our bodies. Free radicals roam the body and damage the genetic material of cells, which may lead to cancer development. They can also damage protein and fat molecules in our cells. Every cell in our body has defense mechanisms against free radicals, including a system of enzymes and antioxidants that act as scavengers, mopping up free radicals before they cause harm. Without continuous antioxidant protection, our cells would not survive. Dietary antioxidants like beta-carotene (and vitamins E and C) provide the body with extra ammunition against free radicals. You'll read more about the effect of beta-carotene in the "Vitamins and Minerals" section below.

The protective effects of fruits and vegetables have not been replicated, however, in studies focussing on isolated antioxidants such as beta-carotene or vitamin C supplements. We are learning that there's more to fruits and vegetables than vitamins, minerals, and fibre. Plant foods also contain thousands of phytochemicals, naturally occurring compounds that act as antioxidants and natural antibiotics, and inhibit cancer development. Experts believe that phytochemicals play a unique role in health and that they probably work together with vitamins and minerals in the food. That's probably why we don't see the same disease prevention in studies using supplements—it's the *whole food* that seems to be important.

Despite our knowledge that these foods are good for us, many of us still don't manage to get our recommended daily 5 to 10 servings. We say we don't have time. We grab a bagel instead of an apple. Or we throw together pasta with tomato sauce instead of eating a salad with a baked potato. Some people just don't like vegetables. Maybe you think that a strawberry cereal bar counts as a fruit serving. Or when it comes right down to it, we'd rather have French fries instead of a bowl of steamed spinach.

Well, now it's time to make sure you get at least 5 to 10 servings of fruits and vegetables each day. Aim to eat at least three different coloured fruits and three different coloured vegetables daily. Try these tricks to sneak them into your diet:

- Buy pre-chopped and washed vegetables at the supermarket. Try baby carrots, broccoli and cauliflower florets, or "salad in a bag." These veggies are ready to be thrown into the microwave, steamer, or your salad bowl.
- Pick up fresh fruit or raw veggies from the salad bar at your local supermarket.
- Grab a can of vegetable juice instead of diet Coke at lunch.
- Order salad at lunch (ask for your dressing on the side).

- For a nutrient boost, use romaine and other dark green lettuces when making salad (I've always referred to iceberg as the "polyester of lettuces"!).
- When you order a sandwich, make sure to ask for tomatoes, cucumbers, and lettuce. When making a sandwich, try spinach leaves as a change from lettuce.
- Add quick cooking greens like spinach, kale, rapini, or Swiss chard to soups and pasta sauces.
- Fortify soups, pasta sauces, and casseroles with grated zucchini and grated carrot.
- Bake (or microwave) a sweet potato for a change from rice or pasta.
- Add slices of lemon, lime, or orange to water for flavour and a little vitamin C.
- Enjoy chocolate cake? Top it with a few spoonfuls of strawberries.
- Replace that cereal bar with two pieces of fruit.

RESEARCH FILE

Antioxidant all stars

An American research team has measured the ability of fresh produce to provide antioxidant protection, that is, to protect cells from harmful free radical molecules. They compared fruits and vegetables to vitamin C and E supplements. Guess what? Most fruits and vegetables outperformed the supplements by a long shot. Here are the real winners ranked according to antioxidant performance:

Vegetables
1. kale
2. beets
3. red peppers
4. broccoli
5. spinach
6. red grapes
7. potato
8. sweet potato
9. corn

Fruits
1. blueberries
2. strawberries
3. plums
4. oranges
5. red grapes
6. kiwi
7. white grapes
8. apples, tomatoes, bananas, pears

FIBRE AND WHEAT BRAN

Although the research is preliminary, there is evidence to suggest that a high fibre intake may offer protection from breast cancer. When Toronto researchers looked at the findings from 12 controlled studies, they found that 20 grams of fibre per day was associated with a modest, but significant, lower risk of developing breast cancer.

One way fibre may help is by binding to estrogen in the intestine and causing it to be excreted in the stool. Every day our intestines reabsorb estrogen from bile, a compound that your liver manufactures and that your gall bladder releases into your intestines. Bile is needed to digest fat. If dietary fibre can attach itself to estrogen and facilitate its removal from the body, your body has to take estrogen out of the bloodstream to make more bile. The net result—a lower level of circulating estrogen! If you eat a high fibre diet for many years then, you could possibly lower your risk for breast cancer.

Diets high in wheat bran and low in fat do lower blood estrogen levels in premenopausal women. A study from the UCLA School of Medicine found that women who ate a 10 percent fat diet with 25 to 35 grams of fibre each day for two months had significantly lower serum estrogen levels than when they ate their regular diets. A more recent study showed that adding 20 grams of wheat bran to the diet had a significant estrogen lowering effect after one month. Women in this study ate 10 grams of wheat bran daily and achieved a significant reduction in estrogen levels after two months.[16]

High fibre diets, because they are high in plant foods, also tend to be higher in antioxidant vitamins and lower in fat, both factors that might protect against breast cancer. People who eat plenty of fibre also tend to maintain a healthy weight. There are many possible explanations for fibre's protective effect, all of which may be true. The studies do suggest, however, that dietary fibre works best if you follow a low fat diet. So adding a little wheat bran to a diet that's high in fat and low in fruits and vegetables probably won't do you much good. More and more we are learning that health protection comes from a *combination of factors* in the diet—the ideal diet includes many low fat foods, high fibre foods, soy foods, and foods rich in antioxidant nutrients and phytochemicals.

Dietary fibre defined

Dietary fibre is found in plant foods—fruits, vegetables, grains, and legumes. It's the material in plants that cannot be broken down by the human digestive tract. To many people, fibre is synonymous with certain brands of breakfast cereal, thanks to heavy advertising campaigns. But if you rely on one single food to get your fibre, you're shortchanging yourself. That's because dietary fibre comes in two varieties, soluble and insoluble. Both types are present in varying proportions in different plant foods, but some foods may be rich in one or the other. And both types of fibre function differently in your body to promote health.

As their name suggests, soluble fibres dissolve in water. Dried peas, beans, and lentils, oats, barley, psyllium husks, apples, and citrus fruits are good sources of soluble fibre. When you consume these foods, the soluble fibres form a gel in your stomach and slow the rate of digestion and absorption. Foods like wheat bran, whole grains, and some vegetables contain mainly insoluble fibres. Although these fibres do not dissolve in water, they do have a significant capacity for retaining water. In this way they act to increase stool bulk and promote regularity. It's wheat bran (containing mostly insoluble fibre) that's been studied the most in relation to breast cancer risk.

How much fibre do you need?

It's estimated that North Americans are getting 11 to 14 grams of fibre each day, only one-half of the daily intake recommended. Most health authorities agree that a daily intake of 25 to 35 grams of dietary fibre is needed to reap its health benefits. To help you sneak more fibre into your diet, see my Nutrition Tip "High Fibre Foods," on page 205. If you're not sure how many grams of fibre you're getting each day, take a look at the fibre content of various foods, below. Note that it's important to gradually build up to consuming 25 to 35 grams of fibre daily. Too much too soon can cause bloating, gas, and possibly diarrhea. When adding fibre to your diet, spread it out over the course of the day. Getting all your fibre at once may reduce the benefits and increase the discomfort. And don't forget that fibre needs water if it's going to do its work. Aim to consume a minimum of one cup (250 millilitres) of water with every high fibre meal and snack.

NUTRITION TIP

High fibre foods

To get the recommended 25 to 35 grams of fibre each day, slowly add new high fibre foods to your diet and replace lower fibre foods you're eating now with choices higher in fibre. All measurements given below refer to amounts after cooking, unless otherwise specified.

FIBRE CONTENT OF HIGH FIBRE FOODS (GRAMS)

Legumes

Black beans, 1 cup (250 ml)	12.0
Chickpeas, 1 cup (250 ml)	6.1
Kidney beans, 1 cup (250 ml)	6.7
Lentils, 1 cup (250 ml)	8.4
Pinto beans, 1 cup (250 ml)	14.0

Nuts

Almonds, 1/2 cup (125 ml)	5.0
Peanuts, 1/2 cup (125 ml)	6.0

Cereals

100% bran cereals, 1/2 cup (125 ml)	10.0
Bran Flakes, 1 cup (250 ml)	5.0
Corn Bran, 1 cup (250 ml)	7.6
Bran Buds, 1/3 cup (75 ml)	13.0
Red River Cereal, 1 cup (250 ml)	5.0
Shreddies, 1 cup (250 ml)	4.0

Bread and grains

Bran muffin, 1 medium	2.5
Pita pocket, whole wheat, 1	4.5
Whole wheat bread, 100%, 2 slices	3.0
Pasta, whole wheat, 1 cup (250 ml)	6.0
Rice, brown, 1 cup (250 ml)	2.5
Wheat bran, 1 tbsp. (15 ml)	1.2

Fruits (raw unless otherwise specified)

Apple, 1 medium with skin	3.5
Apricots, dried, 1/2 cup (125 ml)	6.0
Blackberries, 1/2 cup (125 ml)	3.5
Figs, 3 dried	5.0
Pear, 1 medium with skin	4.7
Prunes, 3 dried	4.0
Orange, 1 medium	2.6
Raisins, 1/2 cup (125 ml)	7.5

Vegetables

Broccoli, 1/2 cup (125 ml)	2.0
Brussels sprouts, 1/2 cup (125 ml)	2.5
Carrots, 1/2 cup (125 ml)	2.5
Green peas, 1/2 cup (125 ml)	4.0
Lima beans, 1/2 cup (125 ml)	4.8
Sweet potato, mashed, 1/2 cup (125 ml)	4.0

YOGURT AND FERMENTED MILK

The last time you sat down to a bowl of yogurt you probably didn't think you might be staving off breast cancer. One Dutch study in which researchers compared the diets of women with breast cancer to the diets of women free of the disease showed that women who ate a low fat diet with plenty of fibre and fermented milk products (the equivalent of 1.5 glasses daily) had a 50 percent lower risk of developing breast cancer than women who did not use fermented milk products regularly. Another study found that fermented milk inhibited the growth of breast cancer cells in the laboratory.[17] Once in our intestinal tract, the bacteria in these foods can produce active compounds that suppress the growth of other microbes that produce cancer-causing substances.

These so called friendly bacteria are known collectively as lactic acid bacteria and include *Lactobacillus acidophilus, Lactobacillus bulgaricus, Lactobacillus casei, Streptococcus thermophilus,* and the many strains of *Bifidobacteria.* The human digestive tract contains hundreds of strains of bacteria, making up what is called the normal intestinal flora. Among the intestinal flora are the lactic acid bacteria. They inhibit the growth of unfriendly, or disease causing, bacteria by producing lactic acid and anti-bacterial substances that suppress their growth, and by preventing unfriendly bacteria from attaching themselves to the intestinal walls. When you take a broad spectrum antibiotic, you end up killing both the disease causing bacteria and the friendly ones. Fermented milk products become even more important when you're on a course of antibiotics.

Fermented milk products actually have a long history of medical use. Records show that foods like yogurt and kefir (a drink made by adding live bacteria to milk) were used by sixteenth-century doctors to treat intestinal infections. Today scientists are learning that these friendly bacteria may do a whole lot more than keep our intestinal tract healthy. In addition to possible cancer prevention, lactic acid bacteria can help stimulate the immune system, lower blood cholesterol, treat candida yeast infections, and speed recovery from diarrhea.

Adding fermented milk products to your diet

Lactic acid bacteria in fermented milk products and supplements will exert their health effects only if they reach the intestines in sufficient numbers. That means you must consume adequate "doses" of live bacteria. Experts generally recommend consuming between one and ten billion living, healthy bacterial cells daily. The amount of live bacteria in a three-quarter cup (175-millilitre) container of yogurt ranges from 175 million to 17,500 million. During storage, these bacteria may die by a factor of 10 to 100. In Canada, all commercial yogurts are made using *Lactobacillus bulgaricus* and *Streptococcus thermophilus.* Some manufacturers add other strains such as some of the *Bifidobacteria, Lactobacillus acidophilus,* and *Lactobacillus casei.* To begin reaping the health benefits of probiotics, include one serving of yogurt in your daily diet. If you're a little more adventurous you might try kefir or sweet acidophilus milk, two fermented milk beverages available in many supermarkets.

Choosing a probiotic supplement

The term "probiotic" literally means "to promote life." As you might have guessed, it refers to living organisms which, upon ingestion in certain numbers, improve the microbial balance in the intestines and exert health benefits. In this sense, yogurt is considered a probiotic food. If you don't eat dairy products, probiotic capsules or tablets are a good alternative. In fact, many natural health experts believe that taking a high quality probiotic supplement is the only way to ensure you're getting a sufficient number of friendly bacteria into your intestinal tract (some of the bacteria in yogurt or a supplement will be killed by acid in the stomach). Even if you do enjoy yogurt or kefir, you might still consider adding a supplement to your daily nutrition regime. Here are a few considerations to keep in mind when choosing a product:

- Buy a product that offers 1 to 10 billion live cells per dose. Taking more than this may result in gastrointestinal discomfort.

- For greater convenience, choose a product that is stable at room temperature and does not require refrigeration. Then you can continue taking your supplement while travelling or at the office. Good manufacturers will test their products to ensure that they maintain their viability over a long period of time. One such product, that has also been used in clinical studies, is called Kyo-Dophilus.

- Know the types and sources of the bacteria in the supplement. Since research has shown that both *Lactobacillus acidophilus* and the various *Bifidobacteria* offer health benefits, a product that contains both types is recommended if you're looking for overall health protection. Many experts believe that human strains of bacteria are better adapted for growth in the human intestinal tract. When choosing a product, you might ask the pharmacist or retailer if the formula contains human or non-human strains.

- Always take your probiotic supplement with food. After a meal, the stomach contents become less acidic due to the presence of food. This allows more live bacteria to withstand stomach acid and reach their final destination in the intestinal tract.

GREEN AND BLACK TEA

A growing body of evidence suggests that tea protects us from certain cancers, including breast cancer. While not all studies that investigate a woman's tea intake find a protective effect against breast cancer, some do. The famous Nurses' Health Study from Harvard found that drinking four or more cups of tea per day (versus one or fewer) was associated with a 30 percent lower risk of breast cancer. Animal studies also show that clear tea, tea with milk, and extracts of tea can suppress or block breast cancer development. And interestingly, a Japanese study discovered that breast cancer patients who drank more green tea before diagnosis had significantly lower recurrence rates and better prognosis than those who didn't.[18] The researchers who did this study now believe that something in green tea may somehow modify the cancer and make it easier to treat.

Like fruits and vegetables, tea is a plant food, harvested from a bush whose scientific name is *Camellia sinensis*. As such, it contains natural chemicals that act as antioxidants. The antioxidants in tea leaves belong to a special class of compounds called catechins. By mopping up harmful free radical molecules in the body, catechins in tea may protect your cells' genetic material from damage.

A study done at Tufts University in Boston compared tea's antioxidant ability to that of 22 different vegetables (including broccoli, onions, garlic, corn, and carrots) and found that 7-ounces (230 millilitres) of green or black tea, brewed for 5 minutes, had an antioxidant power equivalent to that found in the same amount of fruit or vegetable juice.[19]

Types of tea

There are three main types of tea—green, black, and oolong. All three come from the same tea bush, but they are processed differently.

- Green tea. The leaves are allowed to wilt naturally after picking.
- Black tea (a.k.a. the ever popular orange pekoe). The leaves are rolled to break them up and allow air (and thus oxygen) to come into contact with the enzymes in the tea leaves. This contact between the tea enzymes and the oxygen is called fermentation. After fermentation, the leaves are dried.
- Oolong teas. These are made of partially fermented leaves, which gives them a flavour in between that of green and black teas.

In case you're wondering, herbal teas are not made from tea leaves, but from the roots, stems, leaves, and flowers of other plants. They don't have the antioxidant properties of green or black teas. Here are a few tips to help you get a little tea into your diet.

- If you drink coffee in the afternoon, replace it with tea.
- The next time you're at the grocery store, pick up a box of green tea bags or loose leaf green tea. Then, the next time you're having a meal inspired by Asian cuisine at home, you'll be ready to serve it with a pot of green tea. (Of course, you don't have to wait until you're having Asian-type food to enjoy this delicious beverage.)
- Replace all regular and diet soft drinks with tea.
- Enjoy a cup of black tea with your midday snack. Try different flavours—Earl Grey, apricot, and black currant are great.
- The next time you're at your local Starbucks, try chai tea, a spicy hot drink made from tea and spices. You might ask that they add half the amount of syrup as usual—I often find it too sweet.

NUTRITION TIP

Caffeine and tea

Trying to cut back on caffeine *and* lower your odds of breast cancer? Try tea instead of coffee. A cup of tea has one-quarter of the caffeine found in the same amount of coffee, plus you get all its health protecting antioxidants. To reach Health Canada's daily upper caffeine limit of 450 milligrams you'd have to drink 10 to 12 cups of tea a day!

CAFFEINE CONTENT OF COMMON BEVERAGES (MILLIGRAMS)

Black tea, 8 oz. (250 ml)	35
Green tea, 8 oz. (250 ml)	25
Coffee, drip 8 oz. (250 ml)	100 to 175
Cola, 1 can	37

ALCOHOLIC BEVERAGES

So far, I've been mostly recommending that you *add* foods to your diet—foods that the research shows might offer some protection against breast cancer. I realize that alcohol is not a food, but it is a component of many women's diets that needs to be addressed. Unfortunately, that glass of red wine that keeps your heart healthy very likely increases your risk of breast cancer. So likely, in fact, that the diet and cancer experts recommend that women do not drink alcohol. The current recommendations state that if consumed at all, alcoholic drinks should be limited to one per day.

In the late 1970s and early 1980s studies began reporting that breast cancer risk increased with alcohol intake. In a review of 38 studies conducted up until 1992, researchers concluded that having one, two, or three drinks daily all increased the risk of breast cancer. The more alcohol a woman consumed, the higher her risk. Women who drink three alcoholic beverages daily increase the risk of breast cancer by 140 percent as compared to the risk carried by non-drinkers. At three drinks a day the risk is also 20 percent higher than for women who have one drink a day.

We don't fully understand why alcohol increases breast cancer risk. It may be that alcohol weakens breast cells' defenses against carcinogens or it may be that alcohol causes the liver to activate carcinogens. Alcohol may inhibit the ability of cells to repair faulty genes. Alcohol can also influence estrogen levels in the body. In one study, postmenopausal women who consumed two drinks a day had significantly higher blood estrogen levels than women who didn't drink.[20]

Enough evidence has been accumulated that you can conclude that alcohol probably does increase your risk of breast cancer. To help lower your risk, take the following advice to heart:

- If you don't drink alcohol now, don't start.
- If you do drink, aim to consume no more than one drink daily.

- If you need to lower your daily intake, try replacing alcoholic beverages with sparkling mineral water, Clamato or tomato juice, or cranberry and soda.
- You might try cutting out alcoholic beverages on evenings that you are not entertaining or out for dinner. Save your glass of wine or cocktail for social occasions.

MANAGE YOUR WEIGHT

A number of studies have determined that gaining weight after menopause is linked with a higher risk of breast cancer.[21] Obesity may influence breast cancer risk by increasing your circulating estrogen levels—that's because estrogen is produced in body fat cells. If you are overweight, or you have gained some weight since menopause, I strongly advise you to read Chapter 7, "Preventing Weight Gain." On page 78 you are shown how to determine your body mass index. Your body mass index is a key indicator of how your current weight is affecting your health. I also give you plenty of strategies as well as a meal plan (in Appendix 1) to help you achieve a healthy weight.

vitamins and minerals

BETA-CAROTENE AND OTHER CAROTENOIDS

In my discussion of fruits and vegetables, I told you that vegetables high in beta carotene appear to be more protective against cancer than other vegetables. Beta-carotene has two roles in the body. As you read above, it has an antioxidant effect which can help protect our genes from oxidative damage caused by free radicals. But beta-carotene is also converted to vitamin A inside the body. Vitamin A is essential for proper cell growth and development, and also enhances our immunity. Both of these functions of vitamin A may help our body keep cancer at bay.

When all the studies are considered together, beta-carotene does appear to offer some protection from breast cancer. Toronto scientists have estimated that women who get the most beta-carotene in their diets reduce their risk of breast cancer by 15 percent. A diet high in fruits and vegetables rich in beta-carotene might also improve breast cancer survival. Two studies on this topic found that women who consumed more than 8 milligrams of beta-carotene daily had a lower risk of dying from breast cancer than women who got less than 3.5 milligrams each day.

At this time, I am unable to tell you exactly how much beta-carotene you need every day. Unfortunately those studies haven't been done yet. But most experts believe a daily intake of 5 milligrams will offer plenty of antioxidant protection. For the record, one medium sized carrot packs 11 milligrams! You'll get plenty of beta-carotene if you make a point to eat at least two foods from the list below. To boost your beta-carotene, think orange and green!

NUTRITION TIP

Go for green!

Green leafy vegetables are loaded with caretenoids and other antioxidants—and they taste great. Not sure what to do with them? Read on…

Beet greens   When you buy beets, save the greens and eat them too—the leaves of root vegetables have more vitamins and minerals than the roots do! Beet greens are a good source of vitamins A and C, calcium, and iron. They're good in soups, stir-fries, and if tender enough, salad.

Collard greens   In addition to plenty of vitamins and minerals, this cabbage family vegetable contains sulfur compounds that may prevent certain cancers. Stir-fry collards; once cooked, add a dash of roasted sesame oil and a handful of cashews.

Kale   Just one cup (250 millilitres) of this cabbage family green provides more than twice the daily requirements for beta-carotene and vitamin C. Kale is also high in calcium and vitamin E. Steam or stir-fry with other vegetables, or throw chopped kale into soup and simmer. Kale shrinks a lot during cooking; three cups (750 millilitres) raw gives you one cup (250 millilitres) cooked.

Spinach   One-half cup (125 millilitres) of cooked spinach provides plenty of vitamin C, a full day's dose of vitamin A, and plenty of folate, a B vitamin important during pregnancy and for preventing heart disease. One-half cup (125 millilitres) cooked packs more nutrition than one cup (250 millilitres) raw because it contains 2 cups (500 millilitres) of leaves, and heating makes it easier for the body to break down spinach proteins. Steam, braise, or stir-fry with a little garlic. Add a splash of balsamic vinegar at the end of cooking.

Swiss chard   Another great way to get calcium, beta-carotene, vitamin C, and some iron. Use both the leaves and stalks, but add the leaves at the end of cooking—the stalks take longer to soften. Stir-fry with a little olive oil and garlic. Or add lemon juice and Parmesan cheese to cooked Swiss chard. Steamed Swiss chard with a little olive oil and red pepper flakes is great over pasta.

More than 600 different carotenoids exist in plants. While beta-carotene is the most plentiful, other important carotenoids include lutein and lycopene. Researchers are investigating the link between a lutein-rich diet and breast cancer risk. The famous Harvard Nurse's Health Study found that pre-menopausal women who ate five or more servings of high carotenoid fruits and vegetables had a lower risk of breast cancer than women who ate less than two servings daily. In another study of post-menopausal women with breast cancer, researchers discovered that women with higher lutein levels in their blood were more likely to have estrogen-positive breast cancer.[22] As outlined above, breast tumors that contain estrogen receptors are associated with a better chance of survival and better response to hormone treatment.

Dietary carotenoids aren't that well absorbed—our small intestines take in roughly 10 to 30 percent of the amount of these nutrients found in a particular food. Because they are fat-soluble molecules, you'll absorb more if you eat these foods with a little fat. Try a yogurt dip with carrot sticks, a little olive oil in lycopene-rich pasta sauce, or a splash of salad dressing on your roasted red pepper.

To increase your intake of carotenoid-rich fruits and vegetables, try getting five servings (1/2 cup or 125 millilitres each) from a variety of the following foods every day:

CARETENOID-RICH FOODS

Beta-carotene	Lycopene	Lutein
Carrots	Tomatoes	Beet greens
Squash	Tomato sauce	Collards
Sweet potato	Tomato juice	Corn
Red pepper	Grapefruit, red and pink	Kale
Cantaloupe	Guava	Okra
Mango	Watermelon	Red pepper
Nectarine		Romaine lettuce
Papaya		Spinach
Peach		

VITAMIN C

Although the research findings on vitamin C are less consistent than those on beta-carotene, there is evidence to suggest you might need to be getting more in your diet. Nine studies comparing women with breast cancer and those free of the disease found that vitamin C was protective. Women with the most vitamin C in their diet were 27 percent less likely to have breast cancer.[23] The vitamin may keep women healthy by acting as an antioxidant or it may work by enhancing immune system functioning. Vitamin C also plays an important role in collagen synthesis. Collagen is an important tissue found throughout the body, including in the breast—it helps bind cells together, giving the various body structures integrity.

The daily recommended intake of vitamin C for women is 30 milligrams (smokers need double this amount). Refer to page 172 for a list of good food sources of vitamin C and page 173 for information about taking vitamin C supplements.

B VITAMINS

Vitamin B12

Although preliminary, one recent study suggests that a deficiency of vitamin B12 may increase the risk of breast cancer. Harvard researchers reported that post-menopausal women with the lowest B12 levels in their blood had a higher risk of breast cancer than women with much higher levels.[24] It's thought that depleted levels of vitamin B12 can lead to DNA damage.

In the body, vitamin B12 works very closely with folate, an important B vitamin that's needed to synthesize DNA in cells. Folate is needed to activate B12 and vice versa. So without enough B12, your body is unable to use folate and you eventually develop a folate deficiency. That's why you may have heard that it's important to take extra B12 when you take folic acid supplements (folic acid is the name for folate when it's in a pill). Taking plenty of folic acid without additional B12 can hide a B12 deficiency—everything will look normal on a blood test, even though your body is depleted of vitamin B12.

Most B12 deficiencies are caused by impaired absorption, however, not a poor diet. After we consume B12 in our diet, the acid in our stomach helps to release the B12 from food. The vitamin then binds to something called "intrinsic factor" which enables B12 to be absorbed into our bloodstream. Vitamin B12 deficiencies can occur for two reasons:

- Inadequate hydrochloric acid in the stomach, which is common in older adults. Without enough acid, B12 can't be released from food. That means it won't be absorbed into the blood.
- Some people inherit a defective gene for intrinsic factor. They don't produce this necessary factor required for B12 to enter the bloodstream. Regular B12 injections are necessary for these people.

How to get more B12

This vitamin is found exclusively in animal foods. If you eat meat, poultry, and dairy products on a regular basis you're probably okay for B12. The recommended intake for adults is 2.4 micrograms per day. On page 25, you'll find a table outlining various foods and their vitamin B12 content.

For strict vegetarians who eat no animal products and don't drink a fortified soy or rice beverage, I strongly recommend a B12 supplement. As a matter of fact, anyone over the age of 50 should be getting their B12 from supplements or fortified foods. That's because up to one-third of older adults produce inadequate amounts of stomach acid and have lost the ability to properly absorb B12 from food. In this case I recommend a good multivitamin and mineral supplement or a B-complex supplement that contains the whole family of B vitamins.

Folate

If you drink alcohol you might consider getting more folate into your diet. A recent Harvard study found that among women who consumed 15 grams of alcohol per day (about a glass and a half of beer or wine), those with the highest daily intake of folic acid (600 micrograms daily) had a 45 percent lower risk for breast cancer than women with the lowest folate intake (150 to 299 micrograms daily).[25] The correlation between folate intake and breast cancer risk remained even after the researchers took into account the intake of other nutrients, such as beta-carotene or vitamin A. It's thought that alcohol interferes with the transport and metabolism of folate, and may deprive body tissues of this B vitamin, which is essential for DNA synthesis.

So while I told you earlier that drinking alcohol increases the risk of developing breast cancer, this study would suggest that by getting plenty of folate in your diet and taking a folic acid supplement, you might be able to modify that risk. To help you meet the recommended daily intake of 400 micrograms daily, put the following tips into action:

- Eat spinach, asparagus, and artichokes more often. These vegetables have the most folate, with spinach leading the pack.
- One glass of orange juice packs roughly 100 micrograms.
- Use lentils and other legumes in pasta sauces, chilis, and tacos.
- Whole grain breads and cereals are also sources of folate.
- Take a multivitamin and mineral supplement (after reading my first nine chapters you're likely doing this already) or a B-complex supplement.
- If you take a folic acid supplement, be sure to use one that has added vitamin B12.

THE bottom LINE...

Leslie's recommendations for reducing breast cancer risk

1 Reduce your intake of saturated fat (animal fat and hydrogenated vegetable oils) in the following ways: eat no more than three ounces (90 grams) of meat each day; for protein, choose lean poultry, beans, and soy foods most often; when you do eat meat, avoid cooking it well done (unless, of course, you're grilling burgers—to prevent food poisoning, ground beef should be cooked well done); choose lower fat dairy products, including 1% or skim milk, yogurt with 1% milkfat (MF) or less, and cheese with 20% MF content or less.

2 Include monounsaturated and polyunsaturated fats and oils in your diet: to get more omega-3 polyunsaturated fat, eat fish three times a week. Use olive oil and canola oil in cooking and baking and flaxseed oil in salad dressings, or as an addition to already cooked foods.

3 Eat one soy food each day to boost your intake of soy protein and isoflavones. To get plant estrogens called lignans, add one or two tablespoons of ground flaxseed to your daily diet.

4   Eat at least 5 to 10 servings of fruits and vegetables every single day. Make sure 5 of these servings are of foods brimming with carotenoid compounds.

5   Gradually increase your dietary fibre intake to 25 to 35 grams each day. To help lower blood levels of your body's own estrogen, focus on foods rich in wheat bran, such as whole grain breads, 100 percent bran cereals, and whole wheat pasta.

6   Include one probiotic food (fermented milk product) in your diet each day to get more friendly bacteria into your intestinal tract. Try eating one yogurt serving each day as a midday snack or try kefir, a fermented milk product available in most grocery stores. If you don't eat these foods, consider taking a probiotic supplement daily with a meal.

7   Drink more green and black teas for their catechins, natural antioxidant compounds found in tea leaves.

8   Avoid alcoholic beverages. If you do drink, consume no more than one drink each day.

9   Manage your weight before and after menopause.

10 Get more B vitamins into your diet every day, especially folate and vitamin B12. These two vitamins work closely together—folate is needed for DNA synthesis and a deficiency of B12 may increase the risk of breast cancer by leading to damage of DNA molecules. The best food sources of folate include spinach, lentils, orange juice, artichokes, asparagus, and whole grain breads and cereals. If you drink alcoholic beverages, be sure to boost your intake of this B vitamin. Vitamin B12 is found in animal products only—meat, poultry, eggs, and dairy products. Take a multivitamin and mineral supplement daily to ensure you're getting enough B12 and folate. If your multivitamin and mineral is low in B vitamins (less than 5 milligrams of each per dose), consider adding a B-complex supplement to your regime.

Appendix 1

Leslie's total nutrition plan for the menopausal years

This daily nutrition plan is high in fibre and calcium. It provides phytoestrogens from daily servings of soy foods and ground flaxseed. Keep in mind that how you eat throughout the day affects how you feel. To help you boost your metabolic rate and keep energy levels up, I recommend the following:

- Eat your meals 4 to 5 hours apart.
- When meals are eaten more than 5 hours apart, a mid-point snack is strongly recommended.
- Snacks should contain some protein as well as calcium, vitamin D, and antioxidants. To achieve this kind of nutrient profile in your snacks, I recommend that you avoid starchy foods (bagels, crackers, low fat muffins, cereal bars). These foods lack protein and calcium and provide only a short-term energy boost. You'll find my snack suggestions below.

MEAL OPTIONS

Breakfast option 1
- 1 to 2 starchy food servings (whole grain)
- 1 fruit serving (citrus fruit at breakfast to enhance iron absorption from whole grains)
- 1 milk/milk alternative serving
- Ground flaxseed, 1 to 2 tbsp. (15 to 25 ml)
- Green or black tea

Breakfast option 2

- 1 starchy food serving (whole grain)
- 2 fruit servings
- 1 milk/milk alternative serving
- Ground flaxseed, 1 to 2 tbsp. (15 to 25 ml)
- Green or black tea

Breakfast option 3

- 1 protein serving
- 1 to 2 starchy food servings (whole grain)
- 1 fruit serving
- 1 fat serving
- Green or black tea

Mid-morning snack

If breakfast and lunch are 5 to 6 hours apart, eat:
- 1 piece fruit OR 1 milk/milk alternative serving; 2 cups (500 ml) water

If breakfast and lunch are 6 to 7 hours apart, eat:
- 1 piece fruit, 1 milk/milk alternative serving; 2 cups (500 ml) water
  OR
- 1 piece fruit and 1 protein serving; 2 cups (500 ml) water
  OR
- If you're on the go, 1 energy bar containing 14 grams protein (eg. Balance Bar, PR Bar, SoyOne Bar, or Genisoy Bar); 2 cups (500 ml) water

Lunch

- 2 starchy food servings (whole grain)
- 3 protein servings
- 1 to 2 vegetable servings
- 2 fat/oil servings
- 2 cups (500 ml) water

Mid-afternoon snack

If lunch and dinner are 5 to 6 hours apart:

- 1 fruit serving OR 1 milk or milk alternative serving; 2 cups (500 ml) water

If lunch and dinner are 6 to 7 hours apart:

- 1 fruit serving and 1 milk/milk alternative serving; 2 cups (500 ml) water
  OR
- 1 fruit serving and 1 protein serving; 2 cups (500 ml) water
  OR
- If you're on the go, 1 energy bar with 14 grams protein; 2 cups (500 ml) water

Dinner

- 3 to 5 protein servings
- 0 to 2 starchy food servings (whole grain)
- 1 green vegetable serving
- 2 other vegetable servings
- 2 fat/oil servings
- 2 cups (500 ml) water

Evening snack (optional)

- 1 milk/milk alternative serving

MEAL IDEAS

Breakfast ideas

- 1 cup (250 ml) 100 % bran cereal OR 1 1/2 cups (375 ml) whole grain flake cereal. *(Choose a cereal with at least 4 grams fibre per serving.)*
- 1 tbsp. (15 ml) ground flaxseed, sprinkled over cereal
- 1 cup (250 ml) skim or 1% milk OR 1 cup (250 ml) low fat fortified soy beverage
- 3/4 cup (175 ml) unsweetened citrus juice OR 1 cup strawberries
- Green or black tea
  OR

- 1 cup (250 ml) cooked oatmeal or Red River cereal, made with skim or 1% milk instead of water.
- 2 tbsp. (25 ml) ground flaxseed and 2 tbsp. (25 ml) raisins, added to cereal
- 1/2 cup (125 ml) low fat vanilla flavoured yogurt, as cereal topping
- 3/4 cup (175 ml) calcium fortified orange juice or grapefruit juice
- Green or black tea

  OR
- 2 whole wheat toaster waffles
- 1 cup (250 ml) fresh fruit or berries, 3/4 cup (175 ml) low fat vanilla flavoured yogurt, and a drizzling of maple syrup as waffle topping
- 3/4 cup (175 ml) calcium fortified orange juice or grapefruit juice
- Green or black tea

  OR
- Blender smoothie: 1 cup (250 ml) low fat calcium fortified soy beverage, 1 small banana, 1/2 cup (125 ml) orange juice or handful of frozen berries, and 1 to 2 tbsp. (15 to 25 ml) ground flaxseed
- 1 slice whole grain or rye toast with 1 tbsp. (15 ml) sugar reduced fruit jam
- Green or black tea

  OR
- 1 hard boiled or poached egg OR 1 oz. low fat cheese
- 2 slices whole grain or rye toast
- Sugar reduced fruit jam
- 1 cup fruit salad or 1 piece fruit
- 1 cup (250 ml) water
- Green or black tea

Mid-morning snack
- 1 apple and/or 3/4 cup (175 ml) low fat yogurt
- 2 glasses (500 ml) water

Lunch ideas

- Sandwich on two slices of whole grain bread, with 3 oz. (90 g) turkey or chicken breast, 2 tsp. (10 ml) light mayonnaise, and romaine lettuce leaves and sliced tomato.
- Handful of baby carrots or side salad with seasoned rice vinegar
- 2 glasses (500 ml) water

OR

- 1 1/2 cups (375 ml) hearty bean soup
- 4 whole grain crackers or 1/2 whole wheat pita
- Green or spinach salad with 1 tbsp. (15 ml) mixed nuts
- 4 tsp. (20 ml) salad dressing
- 2 glasses (500 ml) water

OR

- Large green or spinach salad
- 4 ounces (120 g) or 1 can tuna or salmon packed in water
- 4 tsp. (20 ml) salad dressing
- 1 whole grain or rye roll
- 2 glasses (500 ml) water

OR

- 1 cup (250 ml) vegetable soup
- Add 1/2 cup (125 ml) cubed firm tofu when heating soup
- Toasted vegetable sandwich on 2 slices whole grain bread (tomato, cucumber, fresh basil leaves, spread with goat cheese)
- 2 glasses (500 ml) water

OR

- 1 cup (250 ml) canned beans (try kidney or black beans) heated with 2 tbsp. (25 ml) water, chili powder, and other spices as desired. Place on 8-inch (20-cm) whole wheat tortilla and top with chopped green pepper, tomato, lettuce, grated cheese, salsa
- 2 glasses (500 ml) water

Mid-afternoon snack ideas

- Blender smoothie: 1 cup (250 ml) low fat calcium fortified soy beverage, 1/2 small banana, and handful of frozen strawberries or blueberries
  OR
- 1 piece fruit and 2 tbsp. (25 ml) roasted soy nuts
- With either snack: 2 glasses (500 ml) water

Dinner ideas

- 5 oz. (150 g) grilled or baked salmon filet, baked in foil with lemon juice, garlic, and chopped fresh dill
- 1/2 to 1 cup (125 to 250 ml) brown rice
- Stir-fried broccoli, red pepper, mushrooms, and slivered almonds, stir-fried in chicken or vegetable broth to prevent sticking
- 2 glasses (500 ml) water
  OR
- Omelet made with 1 whole egg and 4 egg whites (these can be Pure Egg Whites, available at grocery stores)
- Add fresh basil leaves and crumbled goat cheese, or try grated cheddar, chopped green onion, and salsa
- 1 whole grain roll or slice of toast
- Green salad
- 4 tsp. (20 ml) salad dressing
- 2 glasses (500 ml) water
  OR
- 3 oz. (90 g) roasted pork tenderloin, brushed with hoisin sauce, or, if you have more time, marinate in soy sauce, garlic, and chopped ginger then bake at 375 degrees Fahrenheit (190 degrees Celsius) for 30 minutes
- 1/2 cup (125 ml) roasted new potatoes with 1 tsp. (5 ml) olive oil, salt, and herbs
- Steamed vegetables (1 orange and 1 green)
- 2 glasses (500 ml) water

OR

- 1 to 1 1/2 cups (250 to 375 ml) vegetarian chili (homemade with assorted canned beans tastes great)
- 1 small whole wheat tortilla
- 2 cups (500 ml) green salad
- 4 tsp. (20 ml) salad dressing
- 2 glasses (500 ml) water

OR

- 5 oz. (150 g) baked white fish (eg. halibut, swordfish, or sea bass); marinate for 30 minutes with a Japanese-style dressing or brush with hoisin sauce and bake at 425 degrees Fahrenheit (220 degrees Celsius) for 10 to 14 minutes or until done
- Stir-fried collard greens; at the end of cooking add 1 tsp. (5ml) roasted sesame oil and some cashew nuts
- 1/2 cup (125 ml) yam/sweet potato mashed with 2 tbsp. (25 ml) orange juice
- 2 glasses (500 ml) water

OR

- 1 cup (250 ml) cooked whole wheat pasta
- 3/4 cup (175 ml) tomato pasta sauce
- Add 2/3 cup (150 ml) Yves Veggie Cuisine Veggie Ground Round or 2/3 cup (150 ml) white kidney beans to sauce (Yves Cuisine soy products are sold in the produce section of the grocery store)
- Green salad
- 4 tsp. (20 ml) salad dressing
- 2 glasses (500 ml) water

Dessert or evening snack

- 3/4 cup (175 ml) low fat yogurt with added fruit
- 1 tbsp. (15ml) ground flaxseed, mixed into yogurt

YOUR DAILY AND WEEKLY SUPER NUTRITION PLAN CHECKLISTS

Post this list somewhere that's easily visible in your kitchen. After a few weeks of making sure you've fulfilled these requirements, you'll find you've developed a new and healthier set of eating habits.

Your daily checklist

Foods

☐   I soy food serving

☐   2 milk or milk alternative servings

☐   I calcium-rich vegetable

☐   I dark green vegetable

☐   I citrus fruit

☐   I to 2 tbsp. (15–25 ml) ground flaxseed

☐   Flaxseed oil, walnut oil, or nuts

Beverages

☐   8 or more glasses of water

☐   I cup (250 ml) green or back tea

☐   No more than I alcoholic drink

Supplements

☐   Multivitamin/mineral

☐   Vitamin E, 400 or 800 IU

☐   Vitamin C, 500 mg

☐   Calcium citrate with vitamin D and magnesium, 300 to 350 mg

Your weekly checklist

Foods

☐   Fish, 3 times weekly

☐   Nuts, 3 to 5 times weekly

☐   Dessert or other "treat," once weekly

Beverages:

☐   Alcoholic drinks, no more than 7 weekly

Leslie's meal plan for healthy weight loss

BREAKFAST
Every morning, choose among the following breakfast menus:

Breakfast option 1
- 1/2 cup (125 ml) 100% bran cereal OR 1cup (250 ml) whole grain cereal *(choose a cereal with at least 4 grams fibre per serving)*
- 1 cup (250 ml) 1% or skim milk or fortified soy beverage
- 3/4 cup (175 ml) calcium fortified orange juice or 1 piece citrus fruit
- Water
- Vitamin supplements

Breakfast option 2
- 2 slices whole wheat toast with 2 tsp. (10 ml) sugar reduced jam or honey
- 3/4 cup (175 ml) low fat yogurt (fruit bottom okay) or 1 medium sized skim milk latte
- 3/4 cup (175 ml) calcium fortified orange juice or 1 piece fruit
- Water
- Vitamin supplements

Breakfast option 3
- 1 cup (250 ml) cooked oatmeal, Red River or Cream of Wheat cereal *(to boost the nutritional content of your hot cereal, add ground flaxseed, wheat germ, or 2 tbsp. (25 ml) dried fruit—cherries, cranberries, raisins)*
- 3/4 cup (175 ml) plain or vanilla flavoured low fat yogurt or 1 cup (250 ml) fortified soy beverage (or milk)
- 3/4 cup (175 ml) calcium fortified orange juice
- Vitamin supplements

Breakfast option 4
- Soy breakfast smoothie (see recipe, above, on page 222)
- Water and vitamin supplements

MID-MORNING SNACK

Have a mid-morning snack if you take lunch more than five hours after breakfast. Choose one of the following:

- 3/4 cup (175 ml) 1% milkfat yogurt
- 1/4 cup (50 ml) soy nuts
- 1 piece fruit

LUNCH

Your lunch options are as follows:

Lunch option 1

- Sandwich on rye, pumpernickel, whole wheat, or pocket pita filled with 2 to 3 oz. (60 to 90 g) lean protein: turkey, chicken breast, or tuna with low fat mayo
- 2 tsp. (10 ml) mayonnaise or 4 tsp. (20 ml) salad dressing if desired
- 1 vegetable serving (baby carrots, vegetable soup, green salad, vegetable juice)
- Water

Lunch option 2

- 3 oz. (90 g) grilled chicken breast or 3 oz. (90 g) tuna or 3/4 cup (175 ml) cottage cheese
- Large green salad
- 4 tsp. (20 ml) salad dressing or 2 tsp. (10 ml) olive or flaxseed oil
- 1 whole grain roll
- Water

Lunch option 3

- Veggie burger made with soy protein (not a "grain" burger)
- Whole wheat roll or 1/2 whole wheat pita pocket
- Mustard, relish, sliced vegetables
- Green salad with 4 tsp. (20 ml) salad dressing
- Water

Lunch option 4

- 1 cup (250 ml) cooked pasta with tomato sauce and 3 oz. (90 g) seafood or chicken
- Large green salad
- 4 tsp. (20 ml) salad dressing
- Water

MID-AFTERNOON SNACK

Have a mid-afternoon snack if you take dinner more than five hours after lunch. Choose one of the following:

- 1 piece of fruit and 3/4 cup (175 ml) low fat yogurt
- 1 piece fruit and 2 tbsp. (25 ml) roasted soy nuts
- 1 energy bar (look for a bar containing 14 grams of protein and about 200 to 250 calories; try Balance Bar, PR Bar, or Genisoy Bar)

DINNER

I've handled the dinner section a little differently than the others. I'll start by outlining "Your Basic Dinner," and then go on to give you a few menu options that fit the basic pattern.

Your basic dinner

- 4 to 5 oz. (120 to 150 g) baked or grilled poultry, lean meat, fish, or seafood
- NO STARCHY FOODS
- 1–2 cups (250–500 ml) vegetables: aim for at least two different vegetables
- 2 tsp. (10 ml) oil or 4 tsp. (20 ml) salad dressing
- Water

Dinner option 1

- Large green salad
- 1 can tuna (packed in water, drained) OR 1 grilled chicken breast
- 4 tsp. (20 ml) salad dressing
- Water

Dinner option 2

- Omelet made with 1 whole egg* and Pure Egg Whites *(sold right beside the eggs in the grocery store; look for the light blue package)* OR make your omelet with 4 egg whites and add vegetables, 2 tbsp. (30 ml) grated low fat cheese, salsa
- Vegetables steamed, or large green salad
- 4 tsp. (20 ml) salad dressing or 1 tsp. (5 ml) oil/margarine

Try omega-3 eggs, available in all grocery stores

Dinner option 3

- 5 oz. (150 g) baked salmon fillet *(wrap in foil with lemon juice and fresh chopped dill; bake at 400 degrees Fahrenheit (200 degrees Celsius) for 25 to 30 minutes)*
- Plenty of steamed vegetables and/or green salad
- 4 tsp. (20 ml) salad dressing
- Water

Dinner option 4

- 4 oz. (120 g) roasted pork tenderloin *(Brush with hoisin sauce; bake at 375 degrees Fahrenheit (190 degrees Celsius) for 30 minutes)*
- Plenty of steamed vegetables and/or salad
- 4 tsp. (20 ml) salad dressing or 1 tsp. (5 ml) oil
- Water

Dinner option 5

- 4 oz. (120 g) grilled lean beef
- Large green salad and/or steamed vegetables
- 4 tsp. (20 ml) salad dressing or 1 tsp. (5 ml) oil
- Water

Dinner option 6

- 5 oz. (150 g) white fish—halibut, swordfish, sea bass *(Marinate with your favourite dressing or brush with hoisin sauce; bake at 425 degrees Fahrenheit (220 degrees Celsius) for 10 to 14 minutes)*
- Plenty of steamed or stir-fried vegetables or salad
- Water

Daily food intake targets

If you follow the meal plan outlined above you will meet the daily food intake targets given below. In my opinion, maintaining your daily food intake at these target levels is essential for maintaining health while losing weight. In addition, these targets are your guide to lifelong healthy eating patterns. Refer to Appendix 2 for a detailed list of serving sizes.

- Protein foods, daily intake target: *6 to 8 servings*
- Starchy foods, daily intake target: *3 to 4 servings*
- Vegetables, daily target intake: *3 or more servings*
- Fruit, daily intake target: *3 servings*
- Milk products and milk alternatives, daily target intake: *2 to 3 servings*
- Fats and oils, daily target intake: *3 to 4 servings*

appendix 2

what's a serving?

Wondering what constitutes a serving of a particular food? Here's a list of serving sizes for the foods we most commonly eat—use it to help you keep on track with your daily portions. Note that except where noted otherwise, all serving sizes refer to measures *after* cooking.

PROTEIN FOODS

Fish, lean meat, poultry	1 oz. (30 g)
Egg, whole	1
Egg whites	2
Legumes (beans, chickpeas, lentils)	1/3 cup (75 ml)
Soy nuts	2 tbsp. (25 ml)
Tempeh	1/4 cup (50 ml)
Tofu, firm	1/3 cup (75 ml)
Texturized vegetable protein	1/3 cup (75 ml)
Veggie dog, small	1

STARCHY FOODS

Whole grain bread	1 slice
Bagel, regular size	1/4
Roll, large	1/2
Pita pocket	1/2
Tortilla, 6 inch (15 cm)	1
Cereal, flake type	3/4 cup (175 ml)

Cereal, 100% bran	1/2 cup (125 ml)
Cereal, hot	1/2 cup (125 ml)
Crackers, soda	6
Corn niblets	1/2 cup (125 ml)
Popcorn, plain	3 cups (750 ml)
Grains (millet, barley, quinoa, etc.)	1/2 cup (125 ml)
Pasta	1/2 cup (125 ml)
Rice	1/3 cup (75 ml)

VEGETABLES

Vegetables, cooked or raw	1/2 cup (125 ml)
Vegetables, leafy green	1 cup (250 ml)

FRUIT

Fruit, whole	1 piece
Fruit, small (plums, apricots)	4 pieces
Fruit, cut up	1 cup (250 ml)
Berries	1 cup (250 ml)
Juice, unsweetened	1/2 to 3/4 cup (125 to 175 ml)

MILK PRODUCTS AND MILK ALTERNATIVES

Milk	1 cup (250 ml)
Yogurt	3/4 cup (175 ml)
Cheese	1.5 oz. (45 g)
Rice beverage, fortified	1 cup (250 ml)
Soy beverage, fortified	1 cup (250 ml)

FATS AND OILS

Butter, margarine, mayonnaise	1 tsp. (5 ml)
Nuts, seeds	1 tbsp. (15 ml)
Peanut and nut butters	1.5 tsp. (7 ml)
Salad dressing	2 tsp. (10 ml)
Vegetable oil	1 tsp. (5 ml)

appendix 3

soy food recipes

Following is a collection of recipes that get my clients enjoying soy foods. I hope you enjoy them too.

BREAKFAST

Breakfast shake with tofu
From the low fat kitchen of my friend and fellow dietitian, Sandi Williams.
Serves 1

1 cup	calcium enriched orange juice	250 ml
1	small ripe banana or other fruit that appeals	1
3/4 to 1 cup	soft tofu	(175 to 250 ml)

Blend all ingredients into a smoothie for a quick breakfast.
Optional: *For a nutty flavour add 1 tbsp. (15 ml) ground flaxseed.*

LUNCH AND DINNER

Minestrone soup with soy beans

From Sandi Williams, RD

Serves 8

1 tbsp.	olive oil	15 ml
1	medium onion, chopped	1
2	garlic cloves, minced	2
6 cups	vegetable stock or chicken stock	1.5 l
28 oz.	canned tomatoes, chopped (reserve the juice)	840 g
2	potatoes, cut into cubes	2
2	carrots, diced	2
2 cups	green beans, chopped	500 ml
2 cups	cauliflower, chopped	500 ml
1 cup	dried pasta, shell shaped or fusilli	250 ml
1 can	cooked soybeans, drained and rinsed	1 can
2	zucchini, cubed	2
6 oz. can	tomato paste	180 g can
2 tbsp.	dried basil	25 ml
1 tbsp.	dried oregano	15 ml
1/2 to 1 cup	chopped fresh parsley	125 to 250 ml
1/4 tsp.	ground black pepper	2 ml

Heat the oil in a non-stick pan. Sauté onion and garlic. Cook until softened.

Add vegetable stock, canned tomatoes and juice, potatoes, carrots, green beans, cauliflower. Bring to boil and reduce to simmer 15 minutes. Add pasta, soybeans, zucchini, tomato paste. Simmer for 20 minutes. Add basil, oregano, parsley, and pepper. Cook for another 10 minutes.

Optional: Pesto can be added to taste to the entire soup or to each bowl as served (1 tsp. added to each bowl keeps added fat down); or serve with a sprinkle of parmesan cheese if desired.

Sweet potato soup

Serves 6

2 tsp.	canola oil	10 ml
2	cloves garlic, crushed	2
1	medium onion, chopped	1
1 tsp.	curry powder	5 ml
2 large	sweet potatoes, peeled and chopped	2 large
2 cups	water	500 ml
1	vegetable stock cube, crumbled	1
1 1/2 cups	calcium fortified soy beverage	375 ml

Heat oil in large saucepan. Sauté onion and garlic with curry powder until soft. Add sweet potato, water, and stock cube. Simmer covered for 15 minutes or until vegetables are tender. Cool. Blend or process sweet potato mixture until smooth. Gradually add calcium fortified soy beverage, blending until well combined. Return to saucepan and heat through. Do not boil. Season with salt and pepper to taste. Serve with crusty bread.

Source: So Good Soy Beverage, SoyaWorld

Veggie chili

Serves 4

2 tbsp.	canola oil	25 ml
1	large onion, diced	1
1	red or green pepper, diced	1
1	large carrot, diced	1
2	19 oz. (570 g) cans red kidney beans, drained	2
3	14 oz. (420 g) cans tomatoes	3
2 tbsp.	tomato paste	25 ml
1 tbsp.	crushed dried chilies	15 ml
1 tsp.	chili powder	5 ml

1 tsp.	cumin	5 ml
1 tbsp.	dried oregano	15 ml
1 tbsp.	dried basil	15 ml
	salt & pepper, to taste	
11 oz. pkg.	soy ground round (sold in the produce section of grocery stores)	340 g pkg.

Heat oil in Dutch oven until hot and add onion, pepper, and carrot. Sauté for 6 to 8 minutes, stirring occasionally until partially cooked. Add remaining ingredients except soy ground round. Mix well. Bring to a boil and reduce heat to low. Cook 1 hour. Add crumbled soy ground round. Mix well. Turn off heat and let stand 5 minutes before serving.

This recipe can also be made with texturized vegetable protein (TVP). Rehydrate 1 cup (250 ml) of TVP in an equal amount of boiling water before adding to chili.
Source: Yves Veggie Cuisine

Tofu cutlets
Serves 4

1 lb.	firm tofu	500 g
1/4 cup	lime juice	50 ml
2 tbsp.	soy sauce	25 ml
1 tsp.	sesame oil	5 ml
1 tbsp.	honey	15 ml
1 tbsp.	onion, minced	15 ml
1 tbsp.	garlic, minced	15 ml
1 tbsp.	fresh ginger, minced	15 ml
1/4 tsp.	black pepper	2 ml
1 tbsp.	sesame seeds	15 ml

Slice tofu into 4 pieces lengthwise. Combine all other ingredients except the sesame seeds. Add tofu to the marinade and refrigerate for 2 to 4 hours, turning occasionally. Return dish to room temperature. Preheat oven to 350 degrees Fahrenheit (175 degrees Celsius). Sprinkle tofu with sesame seeds. Bake for 45 minutes.
Source: Try-Foods Canada Ltd.

Hot and sour tofu

Serves 4

1 lb.	firm tofu	500 g
2 tbsp.	canola oil	25 ml
1	leek, trimmed, cut in 1-inch (2.5-cm) pieces	1
2	cloves garlic, thinly sliced	1
1 tbsp.	chopped ginger	15 ml
1 tsp.	Asian hot sauce	5 ml
3 tbsp.	soy sauce	45 ml
2 tbsp.	balsamic vinegar	25 ml
3	green onions, slivered	3

Cut tofu into 1-inch (2.5-cm) cubes. Wipe tofu dry. Heat oil in skillet or wok on high heat. Add leek, garlic, and ginger and stir-fry for 30 seconds or until garlic colours slightly. Add tofu and fry 2 minutes per side or until lightly browned. Stir in hot sauce, soy sauce, and vinegar. Bring to boil, cover pan, and simmer 3 minutes. Sprinkle with green onions. Serve with steamed rice and vegetables.

Source: Lucy Waverman, "On Cooking" column, *The Globe and Mail*

DESSERT

Cinnamon raisin rice pudding
From Sandi Williams, RD
Serves 4

1/3 cup	arborio rice (short grain Italian rice)	75 ml
1/3 cup	raisins	75 ml
2 cups	soy beverage, calcium fortified	500 ml
3 tbsp.	maple syrup or honey	45 ml
1 tsp.	vanilla	5 ml
2 tsp.	butter or margarine	10 ml
1/8 tsp.	nutmeg	1.5 ml
pinch	cinnamon	pinch

Preheat the oven to 275 degrees Fahrenheit (135 degrees Celsius). Mix together all of the ingredients except the cinnamon. Pour into a greased 2-quart (2-litre) baking dish. Bake for 2 hours. Sprinkle with cinnamon. Serve hot or cold.

Variations: Add 1 tsp. (5 ml) grated orange rind or lemon rind or try dried cranberries instead of raisins.

Note: This pudding is absolutely delicious but the maple syrup makes it an unappealing brown colour. If you can't get past the colour, use honey instead.

Angel food cake with chocolate orange sauce
Serves 8
Sauce

10.5 oz. pkg.	silken tofu, rinsed and drained	297 g pkg.
1/4 cup	Dutch Process cocoa	50 ml
1/4 cup	sugar	50 ml
1 tbsp.	Grand Marnier or other orange liqueur	15 ml

Cake

1	prepared angel food cake	1
2	peaches, peeled and cut in thin slices	2

1/2 pint	raspberries, washed	275 ml
3	oranges, cut in sections	3
1 tbsp.	Grand Marnier or other orange liqueur	15 ml
8	fresh mint sprigs for garnish	8

In a blender process tofu, cocoa, sugar, and orange liqueur. Refrigerate. Place prepared angel food cake on a serving platter and set aside. Put prepared fruit in a bowl and sprinkle with liqueur; then spoon around cake on the serving platter. When ready to serve, pour chocolate sauce into a serving pitcher and pour over individual servings. Garnish each serving with a mint sprig.

Source: Adapted from the Ontario Soybean Grower's Marketing Board Tofu Recipe Booklet.

appendix 4

a quick reference guide to vitamins and minerals

Eat right and live well, or so the saying goes. A diet that's low in fat and rich in vegetables, fruit, and whole grains will give you plenty of vitamins and minerals. In fact, your body needs more than 45 such nutrients to stay healthy—and you're most likely to find them in whole, unprocessed, or lightly processed foods. Whole foods also offer many other natural compounds that help your body fight disease, like fibre and phyto- (plant) chemicals.

Yet despite the overload of information available today on the benefits of eating what's good for you, many of us don't get enough vitamins and minerals. If you're on the go, under stress, or you're a haphazard eater, chances are you don't always eat right. In fact, nutrition surveys show that many of us don't get enough of very important nutrients like calcium, iron, and zinc.

Even if you are getting the daily recommended nutrient intake (RNI) of all the major vitamins and minerals, there are certain vitamins you probably should get even more of. Vitamins like C, E, and folate may reduce your risk for cancer, heart disease, and other age related illness when taken in amounts greater than the official RNIs.

RNIS AND RDAS

You're probably familiar with Health Canada's "Recommended Nutrient Intakes" or RNIs. RNIs are single numbers that represent the amount of a nutrient that is needed daily to prevent a deficiency of that nutrient. For example, for adult women the RNI for vitamin C is 30 mg. That's how much is needed to prevent the vitamin C deficiency disease called scurvy.

The RNIs were last updated in 1990 and since then, there have been many advances in our understanding of nutrition's role in the prevention of chronic disease. We are learning how much of a nutrient is needed to reduce the risk of diseases like heart disease and certain cancers, not just how much we need to prevent a deficiency symptom.

As a result, a team of Canadian and American experts, working under the auspices of the National Academy of Sciences in the United States, is currently in the process of revising the RNIs. The new recommendations will be made for all North Americans. In the new guidelines, called dietary reference intakes, the term RNI will be replaced by the term recommended dietary allowance (RDA).

Revising the RNIs and harmonizing Canadian and American nutrition recommendations is a slow process and we still have a way to go. The first dietary reference intake report was released in 1997 and discussed calcium and all the nutrients with which it has major interactions, including vitamin D, magnesium, phosphorus, and fluoride. That's why when earlier in the book I discuss how much calcium or magnesium you need, I use the term RDA, not RNI.

The second report, on the B vitamins, was released in April 1998. In March/April of 2000 the report on antioxidant nutrients (vitamins C, E, beta-carotene, and selenium) is scheduled for release.

With this information in mind, you'll be able to read and understand the table below without any problems. Recommendations are given for adults.

So to eat a diet that's brimming with protective vitamins and minerals, use the following guide to help you choose the right foods.

FAT SOLUBLE VITAMINS

	What it does	Best food sources	Daily Needs[a]
Vitamin A	Needed for night and colour vision; supports cell growth and development; maintains healthy skin, hair, nails, bones, and teeth; enhances immune system; may help prevent lung cancer	*Vitamin A:* liver, oily fish, milk, cheese, butter, egg yolks *Beta-carotene:* orange and yellow fruits and vegetables; dark green vegetables	Males: 1,000 RE (Retinol Equivalents) Females: 800 RE

	What it does	Best food sources	Daily Needs[a]
Vitamin D	Regulates body calcium levels; needed for calcium absorption; maintains bones and teeth	Fluid milk, fortified soy and rice beverages, oily fish, egg yolks, butter, margarine (also made by body when exposed to sunlight)	Males & Females[b]: 19 to 50: 200 IU 51 to 70: 400 IU Over 70: 600 IU
Vitamin E	Protects cell membranes; enhances immune system; strong antioxidant; needed for iron metabolism	Vegetable oil, margarine, nuts, seeds, whole grains, green leafy vegetables, asparagus, avocado, wheat germ	Males: 9 mg (13 IU) Females: 6 mg (9 IU)
Vitamin K	Essential for blood clotting	Green peas, broccoli, spinach, leafy green vegetables, liver	Males & Females[c]: 60 to 80 mcg

WATER SOLUBLE VITAMINS

	What it does	Best food sources	Daily Needs
Vitamin C	Supports collagen synthesis and wound healing; strengthens blood vessels; boosts immune system; helps body absorb iron; antioxidant	Citrus fruit, strawberries, kiwi, cantaloupe, broccoli, bell peppers, Brussels sprouts, cabbage, tomatoes, potatoes	Males: 40 mg Females: 30 mg (smokers need double the recommended amounts)
B1 (Thiamin)	Needed for energy metabolism; maintains normal appetite and nerve function	Pork, liver, whole grains, enriched breakfast cereals, legumes, nuts	Males[b]: 1.2 mg Females[b]: 1.1 mg
B2 (Riboflavin)	Used in energy metabolism; supports normal vision; maintains healthy skin	Milk, yogurt, cottage cheese, fortified soy and rice beverages, meat, whole grains, enriched breakfast cereals	Males[b]: 1.3 mg Females[b]: 1.1 mg
B3 (Niacin)	Used in energy metabolism; maintains skin, digestive system, and nerve function	Chicken, tuna, liver, peanuts, whole grains, enriched cereals, dairy products, all high protein foods	Males[b]: 16 mg Females[b]: 14 mg

	What it does	Best food sources	Daily Needs[a]
B6 (Pyridoxine)	Needed for protein and fat metabolism; used to make red blood cells; supports brain serotonin production	Meat, poultry, fish, beans, nuts, seeds, whole grains, green and leafy vegetables, bananas, avocados	Males and Females[b]: 1.3–1.7 mg
Folate	Supports cell division and growth; used to make DNA and red blood cells; prevents neural tube defects in newborns; may prevent heart disease	Spinach, lentils, orange juice, asparagus, avocados, whole grains, seeds, liver	Males and Females[b]: 400 mcg
B12 (Cobalamin)	Maintains nerve function; needed to make DNA and red blood cells	All animal foods, fortified soy and rice beverages	Males & Females[b]: 2.4 mcg (adults over 50 should get B12 from a supplement or fortified foods)
Biotin	Used for energy metabolism, fat synthesis, and amino acid and carbohydrate metabolism	Kidney, liver, oatmeal, egg yolk, soybeans, brewer's yeast, clams, mushrooms, bananas	Males & Females[b]: 30 mg
Pantothenic acid	Needed to break down fats, protein, and carbohydrate for energy; used to make bile, red blood cells, hormones, vitamin D	Widespread in foods	Males & Females[b]: 5 mg
Choline	Necessary for fat metabolism and cell membrane structure; building block for acetylcholine, an important chemical for brain and nerve function	Egg yolks, liver, kidney, meat, brewer's yeast, wheat germ, soybeans, peanuts, green peas	Males[b]: 550 mg Female[b]: 425 mg

MINERALS

	What it does	Best food sources	Daily Needs[a]
Calcium	Needed for strong bones and teeth, muscle fortified contraction and relaxation, nerve function, blood clotting; maintains blood pressure	Milk, yogurt, cheese, soy and rice beverages, tofu, canned salmon (with bones), kale, bok choy, broccoli, chard	Males & Females[b]: 24 to 50: 1,000 mg Over 50: 1,200 mg
Magnesium	Involved in bone growth, protein building, muscle contraction, and transmission of nerve impulses	Nuts, legumes, whole grains, leafy green vegetables, meat, poultry, fish, eggs	Males[b]: 420 mg Females[b]: 320 mg
Phosphorus	Maintains strong bones and teeth; used in metabolism; part of genetic material	Dairy products, meat, poultry, fish, egg yolks, legumes	Males & Females[b]: 700 mg
Iron	Needed to transport oxygen to all cells; supports metabolism	Red meat, seafood, poultry, eggs, legumes, whole grains, enriched breakfast cereals	Males: 9 mg Females: 13 mg (after menopause, 9 mg)
Zinc	Crucial for growth and reproduction; used to make genetic material, immune compounds, enzymes; helps transport vitamin A	Oysters, seafood, red meat, poultry, yogurt, whole grains, enriched cereals	Males: 12 mg Females: 9 mg
Iodide	Used to make thyroid hormones which regulate growth, development, and metabolism	Iodized salt, seafood, sea vegetables, plants grown in iodide rich soil	Males & Females: 160 mcg
Copper	Helps the body absorb iron; needed for nerve fibres, red blood cells, connective tissue, and many enzymes	Liver, meat, shellfish, legumes, prunes	Males & Females[c]: 1.5 to 3 mg

	What it does	Best food sources	Daily Needs[a]
Manganese	Part of many enzymes; facilitates cell metabolism	Coffee, tea, legumes, nuts, wheat bran	Males & Females[c]: 2.5 to 5 mg
Molybdenum	Used for metabolism; helps the body mobilize iron stores	Hard drinking water, meat, whole grains, legumes, green leafy vegetables, organ meats	Males & Females[c]: 75 to 200 mcg
Fluoride	Essential in formation of bones and teeth; helps prevent tooth decay	Drinking water (if fluoridated), tea, seafood	Males[b]: 3.8 mg Females[b]: 3.1 mg
Chromium	Helps insulin regulate blood sugar	Brewer's yeast, molasses, mushrooms, whole grains	Males & Females[c]: 50 to 200 mcg
Selenium	Antioxidant; works with vitamin E to prevent cell damage from free radicals	Seafood, meat, organ meats, grains, onion, garlic, mushrooms	Males: 70 mcg Females: 55 mcg
Sulfur	Necessary for body proteins, bones, and teeth; activates enzymes; regulates blood clotting	Meat, organ meats, poultry, fish, eggs, legumes, dairy products	Not established

[a] Recommended Nutrient Intake (RNI) stated for adults over the age of 24 years, unless noted otherwise. From the Scientific Review Committee's *Nutrition Recommendations*, published in Ottawa, Canada in 1990 by Health and Welfare Canada.

[b] New Dietary Reference Intake from Food and Nutrition Board, National Academy of Sciences – Institute of Medicine.

[c] No RNI established. This amount is considered to be safe and adequate.

appendix 5

resources

ASSOCIATIONS

The American Menopause Foundation Inc.
350 Fifth Avenue, Suite 2822
New York, NY, United States of America 10119
Tel: 212-714-2398
Fax: 212-714-1252
www.americanmenopause.org

Founded in 1993, the American Menopause Foundation is an independent non-profit health organization dedicated to providing support and assistance on all issues concerning menopause. Through a newsletter, literature, and educational programs, the foundation provides the latest information on scientific research and other pertinent facts about menopause.

The North American Menopause Society
P.O. Box 94527
Cleveland, Ohio, United States of America 44101-4527
Tel: 440-442-7550
www.menopause.org

This is a non-profit scientific organization devoted to promoting understanding of menopause and improving the health of women through midlife and beyond. You'll find a list of recommended books, newsletters, and web resources as well as referral lists of menopause clinicians in Canada and the United States.

Osteoporosis Society of Canada
33 Laird Drive
Toronto, Ontario, Canada M4G 3S9
Tel: 416-696-2663
Fax: 416-696-2673
Toll-free: (English) 1-800-463-6842 or (French) 1-800-977-1778
www.osteoporosis.ca

Heart and Stroke Foundation of Canada
222 Queen Street, Suite 1402
Ottawa, Ontario, Canada K1P 5V9
Tel: 613-569-4361
Fax: 613-569-3278
To contact your nearest Heart and Stroke Foundation office call,
toll free, 1-888-HSF-INFO (473-4636)
www.hsf.ca

Canadian Cancer Society
National Office
10 Alcorn Avenue, Suite 200
Toronto, Ontario, Canada M4V 3B1
Tel: 416-961-7223
Fax: 416-961-4189
Cancer Information Service: (Toll-free) 1-888-939-3333
www.cancer.ca

Dietitians of Canada
480 University Avenue, Suite 604
Toronto, Ontario, Canada M5G 1V2
Tel: 416-596-0857
Fax: 416-596-0603
www.dietitians.ca

The Dietitians of Canada is an association of food and nutrition professionals committed to the health and well-being of Canadians. Visit the web site to learn about nutrition resources or to find a dietitian in your community.

National Institute of Nutrition
265 Carling Avenue, Suite 302
Ottawa, Ontario, Canada K1S 2E1
Tel: 613-235-3355
Fax: 613-235-7032
www.nin.ca

This private non-profit organization is dedicated to providing leadership in promoting nutrition for the benefit of all Canadians. The NIN serves as a credible source and objective authority on issues related to nutrition, fosters nutrition research and education in Canada and informs nutrition-related public policy deliberations. At the web site you can read about Canadian nutrition news and publications prepared by the Institute.

Canadian College of Naturopathic Medicine
1255 Sheppard Avenue East
North York, Ontario, Canada M2K 1E2
Tel: 416-498-1255
Fax: 416-498-1576
www.ccnm.edu

BOOKS

Before the Change: Taking Charge of Your Perimenopause
Ann Louise Gittleman
New York, NY: HarperCollins Publishers, 1998

CalciYum! Calcium-Rich, Dairy-Free Vegetarian Recipes
David and Rachelle Bronfman
Toronto, ON: Bromedia, 1998

Dr. Susan Love's Breast Book
Susan M. Love, MD, and Karen Lindsey
New York, NY: Addison-Wesley, 1995 (2nd ed.)

Dr. Susan Love's Hormone Book
Susan M. Love, MD and Karen Lindsey
New York, NY: Random House, 1997

Eat for a Healthy Menopause
Elaine Magee
New York, NY: John Wiley and Sons, Inc., 1996

Estrogen: The Natural Way
Nina Shandler
New York, NY: Villard Books, 1997

Good Nutrition for a Healthy Menopause
Louise Lambert-Lagacé, D.T.P
Stoddart Publishing Co. Ltd., 1999

Menopause
Isaac Schiff, MD, with Ann B. Parson
Toronto, ON: Random House of Canada Limited, 1996

Menopause: A Naturopathic Approach to the Transitional Years
Karen Jensen, ND
Toronto, ON: Prentice-Hall Canada Inc., 1999

Menopause Without Medicine, Third Edition
Linda Ojeda, Ph.D.
Almeda, CA: Hunter House Inc. Publishers, 1989

Menopausal Years: The Wise Woman Way
Susun S. Weed
Woodstock, NY: Ash Tree Publishing, 1992

Natural Menopause
Susan Perry and Kate O'Hanlan, MD
Reading, MA: Addison-Wesley Publishing Co. Inc., 1997

Super Nutrition for Menopause
Ann Louise Gittleman
Garden City Park, NY: Avery Publishing Group, 1998

The Osteoporosis Handbook
Sidney Lou Bonnick, MD, FACP
Dallas, TX: Taylor, 1997

Trouble-Free Menopause: Manage Your Symptoms and Your Weight
Judy Marchel, RD and Linda Konner
New York, NY: Avon Books, 1995

BOOKLETS AND NEWSLETTERS

Menopause Handbook
Montreal Health Press Inc.
P.O. Box 1000
Station Place du Parc
Montreal, PQ, Canada H2W 2N1
Published in 1997 by a woman's collective that has produced books on health and sexuality, this 50-page booklet offers good advice as well as insights into a variety of social and political issues which affect the health and well-being of midlife women. Order a copy for $4 by writing or calling 514-282-1171.

A Friend Indeed
Main Floor, 419 Graham Avenue
Winnipeg, MB, Canada R3C 0M3
Tel: 204-989-8028
Fax: 204-989-8029
www.afriendindeed.ca

Published since 1984, this is considered the "grandmother of all menopause newsletters" and is a recommended resource in many books about menopause. Written for women approaching or experiencing menopause, each issue comprises a feature article, letters, research findings, and other news. A subscription for eight 8-page issues costs $30 + GST (Cdn); back issues are also available for a nominal fee.

SOY COOKBOOKS

Tofu Mania: Add Tofu to Your Favorite Dishes for Optimum Health
Brita Housez
Regina, SK: Centax Books, 1999

Tofu and Soyfoods Cookery
Peter Golbitz
Summertown, TN: Book Publishing Company, 1998

The TVP Cookbook
Dorothy R. Bates
Summertown, TN: Book Publishing Company, 1991

notes

INTRODUCTION

1. Ravnikar VA. 1987. Compliance with hormone therapy. *American Journal of Obstetrics and Gynecology* 156:1332–1334.

   ———. 1992. Compliance with hormone replacement therapy: are women receiving the full impact of hormone replacement therapy preventative health benefits? *Womens Health Issues* 2(2):75–80.

   Rabin DS *et al.* 1999. Why menopausal women do not want to take hormone replacement therapy. *Menopause: The Journal of the North American Menopause Society* 6(1):61–67.

I

1. Albertazzi P *et al.* 1998. The effect of dietary soy supplementation on hot flushes. *Obstetrics and Gynecology* 91(1):6–11.

2. Washburn S *et al.* 1999. Effect of soy protein supplementation on serum lipoproteins, blood pressure, and menopausal symptoms in perimenopausal women. *Menopause* 6(1): 7–13.

3. Hochanadel G *et al.* 1999. Soy isoflavone extract ineffective for alleviation of postmenopausal symptoms. Clinical Research Center, MIT. Unpublished.

   Knight DC *et al.* 1999. The effect of Promensil®, an isoflavone extract, on menopausal symptoms. *Climacteric* 2:79–84.

   Baber RJ *et al.* 1999. Randomized placebo-controlled trial of an isoflavone supplement and menopausal symptoms in women. *Climacteric* 2:85–92.

4. Upmalis DH *et al.* 1999. Effect of biochemical parameters of an oral soy extract used in the treatment of vasomotor symptoms in menopausal women. Abstract report presented at The North American Menopause Society 1999 Meeting. Personal Products Company, North Brunswick, New Jersey.

5. Nachtigall L *et al.* 1999. Abstract presented at North American Menopause Society 1999 Meeting. Tufts University, Boston, Massachusetts.

6. Barton DL *et al.* 1998. Prospective evaluation of vitamin E for hot flashes in breast cancer survivors. *Journal of Clinical Oncology* 16(2):495–500.

   Kronenberg, F. 1994. Hot flashes: phenomenology, quality of life, and search for treatment options. *Experimental Gerontology* 29(3/4):319–336.

7. Foster S. 1999. Black cohosh: a literature review. *Herbalgram* 45:35–49.

   Einer-Jensen N *et al.* 1996. *Cimicifuga* and *Melbrosia* lack estrogenic effects in mice and rats. *Maturitas* 25:149–153.

8. Freudenstein J *et al.* 1999. Influence of an isopropanolic aqueous extract of *Cimicifugae racemosa* rhizoma on the proliferation of MCF-7 cells. *Abstracts of the 23rd International LOF-Symposium on Phyto-Estrogens.* University of Gent, Belgium.

9. Stoll W. 1987. Phytopharmacon influences atrophic vaginal epithelium: double-blind study— *Cimicifuga* vs. estrogenic substances. *Therapeuticum* 1:23–31.

   Lehmann-Willenbrock E, Riedel HH. 1988. Clinical and endocrinological examinations concerning therapy of climacteric symptoms following hysterectomy with remaining ovaries. *Zentrallblatt für Gynäkologie* 110(10):611–618.

Düker E-M *et al.* 1991. Effects of extracts from *Cimicifuga racemosa* on gonadotropin release in menopausal women and ovariectomized rats. *Planta Med.* 57:420–424.

2

1. Minister of National Health and Welfare. 1990. Nutrition Recommendations: *The Report of the Scientific Review Committee.*

2. Landolt HP *et al.* 1995. Caffeine intake (200 mg) in the morning affects human sleep and EEG power spectra at night. *Brain Research* 675(1-2):67–74.

    ——. 1995. Caffeine reduces low-frequency delta activity in the human sleep EEG. *Neuropsychopharmacology* 12(3):229–238.

3. ——. 1996. Late-afternoon ethanol intake affects nocturnal sleep and the sleep EEG in middle aged men. *Journal of Clinical Psychopharmacology* 16(6):428–436.

4. Okawa M *et al.* 1990. Vitamin B12 treatment for sleep-wake rhythm disorders. *Sleep* 13(1):15–23.

    Mayer G *et al.* 1996. Effects of vitamin B12 on performance and circadian rhythm in normal subjects. *Neuropsychopharmacology* 15(5):456–464.

5. Mennini T *et al.* 1993. In vitro study on the interaction of extracts and pure compounds from *Valerian officinalis* root with GABA, benzodiazepine and barbiturate receptors. *Fitoterapia* 64:291–300.

6. Lindahl O *et al.* 1989. Double blind study of a valerian preparation. *Pharmacology Biochemistry and Behaviour* 32:1065–1066.

    Leathwood PD *et al.* 1982. Aqueous extract of valerian root improves sleep quality in man. *Pharmacology Biochemistry and Behaviour* 17:65–71.

    ——. 1985. Aqueous extract of valerian root reduces latency to fall asleep in man. *Planta Medica* 51:144–148.

    Vorbach EU *et al.* 1996.Therapie von Insomnien: Wirksamkeit und vertaglichkeit eines Baldrian-Praparates. *Psychopharmakotherapie* 3:109-115.

3

1. Carranza-Lira S *et al.* 1997. Changes in symptomatology, hormones, lipids and bone density after hysterectomy. *International Journal of Fertility and Women's Medicine* 42(1):43–47.

    Crosognani PG et al. Endometrial resection versus vaginal hysterectomy for menorrhagia: long term clinical and quality of life outcomes. *American Journal of Obstetrics and Gynecology* 1997; 177(1):95-101.

2. Wurtman RJ and Wurtman JJ. 1996. Brain serotonin, carbohydrate craving, obesity and depression. *Advances in Experimental Medicine and Biology* 398:35–41.

    Wurtman JJ. 1993. Depression and weight gain: the serotonin connection. *Journal of Affective Disorders* 29(2-3):183–192.

    Christensen L. 1993. Effects of eating behaviour on mood: a review of the literature. *International Journal of Eating Disorders* 14(2):171–183.

    Blum I *et al.* 1992. The influence of meal composition on plasma serotonin and norepinephrine concentrations. *Metabolism* 41(2):137–140.

    Sayegh R *et al.* 1995. The effect of a carbohydrate-rich beverage on mood, appetite, and cognitive function in women with premenstrual syndrome. *Obstetrics and Gynecology* 86(4 pt 1):520–528.

3. Macdiarmid JI and MM Hetherington. 1995. Mood modulation by food: an exploration of affect and cravings in 'chocolate addicts.' *British Journal of Clinical Psychology* 34(pt 1):129–138.

    Di Tomaso E *at al.* 1996. Brain cannibinoids in chocolate. *Nature* 382:677–678.

4. Edwards R *et al.* 1998. Omega-3 polyunsaturated fatty acid levels in the diet and red blood cell membranes of depressed patients. *Journal of Affective Disorders* 48(2–3):149–155.

5. Stoll AL *et al.* 1999. Omega 3 fatty acids in bipolar disorder: a preliminary double-blind, placebo controlled trial. *Archives of General Psychiatry* 56(5):407–412.

6. McCullough A *et al.* 1990. Vitamin B6 status of Egyptian mothers: relation to infant behaviour and maternal-infant interactions. *American Journal of Clinical Nutrition* 51:1067–1074.

    Wyatt KM *et al.* 1999. Efficacy of vitamin B6 in the treatment of premenstrual syndrome: systematic review. *British Journal of Medicine* 318(7195):1375–1381.

7. Linde K *et al.* 1996. St. John's Wort for depression—an overview and meta-analysis of randomized clinical trials. *British Medical Journal* 313:253–258.

Laakmann G *et al.* 1998. St. John's Wort in mild to moderate depression: the relevance of hyperforin for the clinical efficacy. *Pharmacopsychiatry* 31 (suppl.):54–59.

Schellenberg R *et al.* 1998. Pharmacodynamic effects of two different hypericum extracts in healthy volunteers measured by quantitative EEG. *Pharmacopsychiatry* 31 (suppl.):44–53.

8. Kinzler *et al.* 1991. Wirksamkeit eines Kava-Spezial-Extraktes bei Patienten mit Angst-, Spannungs- and Erregungszuständen nicht-psychotischer Genese. *Arzneim Forsch/Drug Research* 41:584–588.

Warnecke G *et al.* 1990. Wirksamkeit von Kawa-Kawa-Extrakt beim klimakterischen Syndrom. *Phytotherapie* 11:81–86.

4

1. Polo-Kantola P *et al.* 1998. The effect of short-term estrogen replacement therapy on cognition: a randomized, double-blind, cross-over trial in post-menopausal women. *Obstetrics and Gynecology* 91(3): 459–466.

2. Sherwin BB. 1998. Estrogen and cognitive functioning in women. *Proc Soc Exp Biol Med* 217(1):17–22.

Yaffe K *et al.* 1998. Estrogen therapy in postmenopausal women: effects on cognitive function and dementia. *Journal of the American Medical Association* 279(9):688–695.

Waring SC *et al.* 1999. Postmenopausal estrogen replacement therapy and the risk of AD: a population-based study. *Neurology* 52(5):965–970.

Baldereschi M *et al.* 1998. Estrogen-replacement therapy and Alzheimer's disease in the Italian Longitudinal Study on Aging. *Neurology* 50(4):996–1002.

Asthana S *et al.* 1999. Cognitive and neuroendocrine response to a transdermal estrogen in post-menopausal women with Alzheimer's disease: results of a placebo-controlled, double-blind, pilot study. *Psychoneuroendocrinology* 24(6):657–677.

3. Smith A *et al.* 1994. Effects of breakfast and caffeine on cognitive performance, mood and cardiovascular functioning. *Appetite* 22(1):39–55.

4. Le Bars PL, *et al.* 1997. A placebo-controlled, double-blind, randomized trial of an extract of *Ginkgo biloba* for dementia. North American EGb Study Group. *Journal of the American Medical Association* 278(16):1327–32.

———. 1988. *Ginkoglides: Chemistry, Biology, Pharmacology and Clinical Perspectives. Volume I.* Barcelona: JR Prous Science.

Braquet P *(ed)*. 1989. *Ginkoglides. Chemistry, Biology, Pharmacology and Clinical Perspectives. Volume II.* Barcelona: JR Prous Science.

Itil TM *et al.* 1996. Central nervous system effects of Gingko biloba, a plant extract. *American Journal of Therapeutics* 3:63–73.

5

1. Sarrel P *et al.* 1998. Estrogen and estrogen–androgen replacement in postmenopausal women dissatisfied with estrogen–therapy. *Sexual behaviour and neuroendocrine responses. Journal of Reproductive Medicine* 43(10):847–856.

Warnock JK *et al.* 1999. Female hypoactive sexual disorder: case studies of physiologic androgen replacement. *Journal of Sex and Marital Therapy* 25(3):175–182.

Simon J *et al.* 199. Differential effects of estrogen-androgen and estrogen-only therapy on vasomotor symptoms, gonadotropin secretion, and endogenous androgen biovailability in postmenopausal women. *Menopause* 6(2):138–146.

2. Brzezinski A *et al.* 1997. Short–term effects of phytoestrogen–rich diet on postmenopausal women. *The Journal of the North American Menopause Society* 4(2):89–94.

Washburn S *et al.* 1999. Effect of soy protein supplementation on serum lipoproteins, blood pressure, and menopausal symptoms in peri-menopausal women. *Menopause* 6(1):7–13.

Baird DD *et al.* 1995. Dietary intervention study to assess estrogenicity of dietary soy among post-menopausal women. *Journal of Clinical Endocrinology and Metabolism* 80(5):1685–1690.

3. Punnonen R and Lukola A. 1980. Oestrogen-like effect of ginseng. *British Medical Journal* 281(6248):1110

4. Balon R. 1999. Ginkgo biloba for antidepressant-induced sexual dysfunction? *Journal of Sex and Marital Therapy* 25(1):1–2.

5. Hirata JD *et al.* 1997. Does dong quai have estrogenic effects in postmenopausal women? A double-blind, placebo-controlled trial. *Fertility and Sterility* 68(6):981–986.

7

1. Reubinoff BE *et al.* 1995. Effects of hormone replacement therapy on weight, body composition, fat distribution and food intake in early post-menopausal women. *Fertility and Sterility* 64(5):963–968.

2. Ludwig DS *et al.* 1999. High glycemic index foods, overeating, and obesity. *Pediatrics* 103(3):E26.

3. Holt SH *et al.* 1995. A satiety index of common foods. *European Journal of Clinical Nutrition* 49(9):675–90.

4. Walker LS *et al.* 1998. Chromium picolinate effects on body composition and muscular per-formance in wrestlers. *Medicine Science and Sports Exercise* 39(12):1730–1737.

   Trent LK and D Thieding-Cancel D. 1995. Effects of chromium picolinate on body composition. *Journal of Medicine and Physical Fitness* 35(4):273–180.

5. Hoeger WW *et al.* 1998. Four-week supplementa-tion with a natural dietary compound produces favorable changes in body composition. *Advances in Therapeutics* 15(5):305–314.

   Grant KE *et al.* 1997. Chromium and exercise training: effects on obese women. *Medicine Science in Sports and Exercise* 29(8):992–998.

6. Colker CM *et al.* 1999. Effects of *Citrus auran-tium* extract, caffeine, and St. John's Wort on body fat loss, lipid levels, and mood states in overweight healthy adults. *Current Therapeutic Research* 60(3):145–153.

7. Heymsfield SB *et al.* 1998. *Garcinia cambogia* (hydroxycitric acid) as a potential antiobesity agent: a randomized controlled trial. *Journal of the American Medical Association* 280(18):1596–1600.

8

1. Cornuz J *et al.* 1999. Smoking, smoking cessation, and risk of hip fracture in women. *American Journal of Medicine* 106(3):311–314.

   Hollenbach KA *et al.* 1993. Cigarette smoking and bone mineral density in older men and women. *American Journal of Public Health* 83(9):1265–1270.

   Egger P *et al.* 1996. Cigarette smoking and bone mineral density in the elderly. *Journal of Epidemiology and Community Health* 50(1):47–50.

2. Grodstein F *et al.* 1999. Postmenopausal hormone therapy and risk of cardiovascular disease and hip fracture in a cohort of Swedish women. *Epidemiology* 10(5):476–480.

   Michaelsson K *et al.* 1998. Variation in the efficacy of hormone replacement therapy in the prevention of hip fracture. Swedish Hip Fracture Study Group. *Osteoporosis International* 8(6):540–546.

   Kiel DP *et al.* 1987. Hip fracture and the use of estrogens in postmenopausal women. The Framingham Study. *New England Journal of Medicine* 317(19):1169–1174.

   Ribot CA *et al.* 1997. Effect of estrogens on bone and other systems and hormonal substitute treat-ment. *Current Opinion in Rheumatology* 9(4):362–369.

   Notelovitz M. 1997. Estrogen therapy and osteo-porosis: principles & practice. *American Journal of Medical Science* 313(1):2–12.

3. Recker RR *et al.* 1999. The effect of low-dose con-tinuous estrogen and progesterone therapy with calcium and vitamin D in elderly women. A ran-domized, controlled trial. *Annals of Internal Medicine* 130(11):897–904.

4. Ravnikar VA. 1987. Compliance with hormone therapy. *American Journal of Obstetrics and Gynecology* 156(5):1332–1334.

   Hammond CB. 1994. Women's concerns with hormone replacement therapy—compliance issues. *Fertility and Sterility* 62(6 Suppl 2):157S–160S.

5. van Staa TP *et al.* 1998. Use of cyclical etidronate and prevention of non-vertebral fractures. *British Journal of Rheumatology* 37(1):87–94.

   Lyritis GP *et al.* 1997. The effect of a modified etidronate cyclical regimen on postmenopausal osteoporosis: a four-year study. *Clinical Rheumatology* 16(4):354–60.

6. Hosking D *et al.* 1998. Prevention of bone loss with Alendronate in postmenopausal women under 60 years of age. *New England Journal of Medicine* 338(8):485–492.

7. Lufkin EG *et al.* 1998. Treatment of established postmenopausal osteoporosis with raloxifene: a randomized trial. *Journal of Bone Mineral Research* 13(11):1747–1754.

8. Alekel Dl *et al.* 1999. Isoflavone-rich soy protein isolate exerts significant bone sparing effect in the lumbar spine of perimenopausal women. Abstract. Third International Symposium on the Role of Soy in Preventing and Treating Chronic Disease.

Schieber MD *et al.* 1999. Dietary soy isoflavones favorably influence lipids and bone turnover in healthy postmenopausal women. Abstract. Third International Symposium on the Role of Soy in Preventing and Treating Chronic Disease.

9. Munger RG *et al.* 1999. Prospective study of dietary protein intake and risk of hip fracture in postmenopausal women. *American Journal of Clinical Nutrition* 69(1):147–152.

Schurch MA *et al.* 1998. Protein supplements increase serum insulin-like growth factor-I levels and attenuate proximal femur bone loss in patients with recent hip fracture. A randomized, double-blind, placebo-controlled trial. *Annals of Internal Medicine* 128(10):801–809.

10. Feskanich D *et al.* 1999. Moderate alcohol consumption and bone density among postmenopausal women. *Journal of Women's Health* 8(1):65–73.

11. Lloyd T *et al.* 1997. Dietary caffeine intake and bone status of postmenopausal women. *American Journal of Clinical Nutrition* 65(6):1826–1830.

Harris SS and B Dawson-Hughes. 1994. Caffeine and bone loss in healthy menopausal women. *American Journal of Clinical Nutrition* 60(4): 573–578.

12. Devine A *et al.* 1995. A longitudinal study of the effect of sodium and calcium intakes on regional bone density in postmenopausal women. *American Journal of Clinical Nutrition* 62(4):740–745.

13. Baran D *et al.* 1990. Dietary modification with dairy products for preventing vertebral bone loss in premenopausal women: a three-year prospective study. *Journal of Clinical Endocrinology and Metabolism* 70(1):264–270.

14. Sakhaee K *et al.* 1998. The effect of calcium citrate on bone density in the early and mid–postmenopausal period: a randomized, placebo-controlled study. Abstract. The Second Joint Meeting of the American Society for Bone and Mineral Research and the International Bone and Mineral Society. Mission Pharmacal Company.

Baran DT *et al.* 1999. A placebo-controlled study of pre-menopausal women: calcium supplementation and bone density. Abstract. Annual Meeting of the American Society for Bone and Mineral Research.

Storm D *et al.* 1998. Calcium supplementation prevents seasonal bone loss and changes in biochemical markers of bone turnover in elderly New England women: a randomized placebo-controlled trial. *Journal of Clinical Endocrinology and Metabolism* 83(11):3817–3825.

Ricci TA *et al.* 1998. Calcium supplementation suppresses bone turnover during weight reduction in postmenopausal women. *Journal of Bone Mineral Research* 13(6):1045–1050.

15. Harris SS and B Dawson-Hughes. 1998. Seasonal changes in plasma 25-hydroxyvitamin D concentrations of young American black and white women. *American Journal of Clinical Nutrition* 67(6):1232–1236.

16. Feskanich D *et al.* 1999. Vitamin K intake and hip fractures in women: a prospective study. *American Journal of Clinical Nutrition* 69(1):74–79.

17. Strause L *et al.* 1994. Spinal bone loss in postmenopausal women supplemented with calcium and trace minerals. *Journal of Nutrition* 124(7):1060–1064.

18. Wolff I *et al.* 1999. The effect of exercise training programs on bone mass: a meta-analysis of published controlled trials in pre- and postmenopausal women. *Osteoporosis International* 9(1):1–12.

Dalsky GP *et al.* 1988. Weight-bearing exercise training and lumbar bone mineral content in postmenopausal women. *Annals of Internal Medicine* (6):824–828.

Pruitt LA *et al.* 1992. Weight-training effects on bone mineral density in early postmenopausal women. *Journal of Bone Mineral Research* 7(2):179–185.

9

1. Heart and Stroke Foundation of Canada. 1995. *Heart Disease and Stroke in Canada, 1995.* Ottawa.

Smurawska LT *et al.* 1994. Cost of acute stroke care in Toronto, Canada. *Stroke* 25(8):1628–1631.

Wingate S. 1995. Quality of life for women after a myocardial infarction. *Heart and Lung* 24(6):467–473.

2. Connelly PW *et al.* 1992. Canadian Heart Health Surveys Research Group. Plasma lipids and lipoproteins and the prevalence of risk for coronary heart disease in Canadian adults. *Canadian Medical Association Journal* 146(11):1977–1987.

Health Canada. 1995. *Canadians and Heart Health: Reducing the Risk.* Ottawa.

La Rosa JC. 1992. Lipids and cardiovascular disease: do the findings and therapy apply equally to men and women? *Women's Health Issues* 2(2):102–111.

Austin MA. 1989. Plasma triglyceride as a risk factor for coronary heart disease: the epidemiologic evidence and beyond. *American Journal of Epidemiology* 129:249–259.

3. Kinosian B *et al*. 1994. Cholesterol and coronary heart disease predicting risks by ratios and levels. *Annals of Internal Medicine* 121:641–647.

4. Kawachi I *et al*. 1994. Smoking cessation and time course of decreased risks of coronary heart disease in middle-aged women. *Archives of Internal Medicine* 154(2):169–175.

    Kawachi I *et al*. 1993. Smoking cessation in relation to total mortality rates in women. A prospective cohort study. *Annals of Internal Medicine* 119(10):992–1000.

5. Kannel WB and DL McGee. 1979. Diabetes and cardiovascular disease. The Framingham Study. *Journal of the American Medical Association* 241:2035–2038.

6. Health Canada. 1995. *Canadians and Heart Health: Reducing the Risk*. Ottawa.

7. Rexrode KM *et al*. 1998. Abdominal adiposity and coronary heart disease in women. *Journal of the American Heart Association* 280(21):1843–1848.

8. Boers GH *et al*. 1985. Heterozygosity for homocystinuria in premature peripheral and cerebral occlusive arterial disease. *New England Journal of Medicine* 313(12):709–715.

    Whincup PH *et al*. 1999. Serum total homocysteine and coronary heart disease: prospective study in middle aged men. *Heart* 82(4):448–454.

    Bots ML *et al*. 1999. Homocysteine and short-term risk of myocardial infarction and stroke in the elderly: the Rotterdam Study. *Arch Intern Medicine* 159(1):38–44.

    Arnesen E *et al*. 1995. Serum total homocysteine and coronary heart disease. *International Journal of Epidemiology* 24(4):704–709.

    Ridker PM *et al*. 1999. Homocysteine and risk of cardiovascular disease among postmenopausal women. *Journal of the American Medical Association* 281(19):1817–1821.

9. Heart and Stoke Foundation. 1999. *Annual Report Card on Canadians' Health*. Toronto.

10. Keys A. 1970. Coronary heart disease in seven countries. *Circulation* Suppl 41:11–1211.

    Stallones RA. 1983. Ischemic heart disease and lipids in the blood and diet. *Annual Reviews of Nutrition* 3:155–185.

    Stamler J. 1979. Population studies pp. 25–88 in Levy RJ *et al* eds. *Nutrition. Lipids and Coronary Heart Disease: A Global View. Nutrition in Health and Disease, Vol. 1.* New York: Raven Press.

11. Hu FB *et al*. 1997. Dietary fat intake and the risk of coronary heart disease in women. *New England Journal of Medicine* 337(21):1491–1499.

    Willett WC *et al*. 1993. Intake of trans fatty acids and risk of coronary heart disease among women. *Lancet* 341(8845):581–585.

    Tavani A *et al*. 1997. Margarine intake and risk of nonfatal acute myocardial infarction in Italian women. *European Journal of Clinical Nutrition* Vol. 51(1):30–32.

12. Rogers AE *et al*. 1986. Chemically induced mammary gland tumors in rats: modulation by dietary fat. *Progress in Clinical Biology Research* 222:255–282.

13. Albert Cm *et al*. 1998. Fish consumption and the risk of sudden cardiac death. *Journal of the American Medical Association* 279(1):23–28.

    Daviglus ML *et al*. 1997. Fish consumption and the 30-year risk of fatal myocardial infarction. *New England Journal of Medicine* 336(15):1046–1053.

    Menotti A *et al*. 1999. Food intake patterns and 25-year mortality from coronary heart disease: cross-cultural correlations in the Seven Countries Study. The Seven Countries Study Research Group. *European Journal of Epidemiology* 15(6):507–515.

14. Hu FB *et al*. 1999. Dietary intake of alpha-linolenic acid and risk of fatal ischemic heart disease among women. *American Journal of Clinical Nutrition* 69(5):890–897.

15. Larsen LF *et al*. 1999. Are olive oil diets antithrombotic? Diets enriched with olive, rapeseed, or sunflower oil affect postprandial factor VII differently. *American Journal of Clinical Nutrition* 70(6):976–982.

    Lindholm LH *et al*. 1992. Risk factors for ischemic heart disease in a Greek population. A cross-sectional study of men and women living in the village of Spili in Crete. *European Heart Journal* 13(3):291–298.

16. De Lorgeril M *et al.* 1999. Mediterranean diet, traditional risk factors, and the rate of cardiovascular complications after myocardial infarction: final report of the Lyon Diet Heart Study. *Circulation* 99(6):779–785.

17. Hu FB *et al.* 1999. A prospective study of egg consumption and risk of cardiovascular disease in men and women. *Journal of the American Medical Association* 281(15):1387–1394.

18. Anderson JW *et al.* 1995. Meta-analysis of the effects of soy protein intake on serum lipids. *New England Journal of Medicine* 333(5):276–282.

    Washburn S *et al.* 1999. Effect of soy protein supplementation on serum lipoproteins, blood pressure, and menopausal symptoms in perimenopausal women. *Menopause* 6(1):7–13.

    Crouse JR *et al.* 1999. A randomized trial comparing the effect of casein with that of soy protein containing varying amounts of isoflavones on plasma concentrations of lipids and lipoproteins. *Archives of Internal Medicine* 159(17):2070–2076.

    Schieber MD *et al.* 1999. Dietary soy isoflavones favorably influence lipids and bone turnover in healthy postmenopausal women. Abstract. Third International Symposium on the Role of Soy in Preventing and Treating Chronic Disease.

    Wilcox JN and BF Blumenthal. 1995. Thrombotic mechanism in atherosclerosis: potential impact of soy proteins. *Journal of Nutrition* 125(3 Suppl):631–638.

19. MacKay S and MJ Ball. 1992. Do beans and oat bran add to the effectiveness of a low fat diet? *European Journal of Clinical Nutrition* 46(9):641–648.

    Braaten JT *et al.* 1994. Oat beta-glucan reduces blood cholesterol concentration in hypercholesterolemic subjects. *European Journal of Clinical Nutrition* 48(7):465–474.

    Uusitupa MI *et al.* 1992. A controlled study of the effect of beta–glucan rich oat bran on serum lipids in hyercholesterolemic subjects: relation to apolipoprotein E phenotype. *Journal of American Coll Nutrition* 11(6):651–659.

    Whyte JL *et al.* 1992. Oat bran lowers plasma cholesterol levels in mildly hypercholesterolemic men. *Journal of the American Dietetic Association* 92(4):446–449.

    Davidson MH *et al.* 1991. The hypocholesterolemic effects of beta-glucan in oatmeal and oat bran. A dose controlled study. *Journal of the American Dietetic Association* 265(14):1833–1939.

Olson BH *et al.* 1997. Psyllium-enriched cereals lower blood total cholesterol and LDL cholesterol, but not HDL cholesterol, in hypercholesterolemic adults: results of a meta-analysis. *Journal of Nutrition* 127(10):1973–1980.

20. Liu S *et al.* 1999. Whole-grain consumption and risk of coronary heart disease: results from the Nurses' Health Study. *American Journal of Clinical Nutrition* 70(3):412–419.

    Jacobs DR Jr. *et al.* 1998. Whole-grain intake may reduce the risk of ischemic heart disease death in postmenopausal women: the Iowa Women's Health Study. *American Journal of Clinical Nutrition* 68(2):248–257.

21. Hu FB *et al.* Frequent nut consumption and risk of coronary heart disease in women: prospective cohort study. <<INCOMPLETE>>

    Lavedrine F *et al.* 1999. Blood cholesterol and walnut consumption: a cross–sectional survey in France. *Preventative Medicine* 28(4):333–339.

22. Sesso HD *et al.* 1999. Coffee and tea intake and the risk of myocardial infarction. *American Journal of Epidemiology* 149(2):162–167.

    Yochum L *et al.* 1999. Dietary flavonoids and risk of cardiovascular disease in postmenopausal women. *American Journal of Epidemiology* 149(10):943–949.

23. Geleijnse JM *et al.* 1999. Tea flavonoids may protect against atherosclerosis: the Rotterdam Study. *Archives of Internal Medicine* 159(18):2170–2174.

    Hertog MG *et al.* 1993. Dietary antioxidant flavonoids and risk of coronary heart disease: the Zutphen Elderly Study. *Lancet* 342(8878):1007–1011.

24. Hankinson SE *et al.* 1995. Alcohol consumption and mortality among women. *New England Journal of Medicine* 332(19):1245–1250.

    Gaziano JM *et al.* Moderate alcohol intake, increased levels of high-density lipoprotein and its subfractions, and decreased risk of myocardial infarction. *New England Journal of Medicine* 329(25):1829–1834.

    Muntwyler J *et al.* 1998. Mortality and light to moderate alcohol consumption after myocardial infarction. *Lancet* 352(9144):1882–1885.

25. Appel LJ *et al.* 1997. A clinical trial of the effects of dietary patterns on blood pressure. *New England Journal of Medicine* 65(Suppl):643S–651S.

26. Rimm EB *et al.* 1998. Folate and vitamin B6 from diet and supplements in relation to risk of coronary heart disease among women. *Journal of the American Medical Association* 279(5):359–364.

27. Nyyssonen K et al. 1997. Vitamin C deficiency and risk of myocardial infarction: prospective study in men from eastern Finland. *British Journal of Medicine* 314(7081):634–638.

Lopes C et al. 1998. Diet and risk of myocardial infarction. A case-control community-based study. *Acta Med Port* 11(4):311-317

Simon JA et al. 1998. Serum ascorbic acid and cardiovascular disease prevalence. *Epidemiology* 9(3):316–321.

28. Gatto LM et al. 1996. Ascorbic acid induces favorable lipid profiles in women. *Journal of the American College of Nutrition* 15:154–158.

Ness AR et al. 1996. Vitamin C status and serum lipids. *European Journal of Clinical Nutrition* 50:724–729.

Bordia A et al. 1980. The effect of vitamin C on blood lipids, fibrinolytic activity and platelet adhesiveness in patients with coronary heart disease. *Atherosclerosis* 35:1810–1817.

Calzada C et al. 1997. The influence of antioxidant nutrients on platelet function in healthy volunteers. *Atherosclerosis* 128:97–105.

29. Stampfer MJ et al. 1993. Vitamin E consumption and the risk of coronary disease in women. *New England Journal of Medicine* 328(20):1444–1449.

Rimm EB et al. 1993. Vitamin E consumption and the risk of coronary heart disease in men. *New England Journal of Medicine* 328(20):1450–1456.

Meyer F et al. 1996. Lower ischemic heart disease incidence and mortality among vitamin supplement users. *Canadian Journal of Cardiology* 12(10):930–934.

Stephens NG et al. 1996. Randomised controlled trial of vitamin E in patients with coronary heart disease. *Cambridge Heart Antioxidant Study* 347(9004):781–786.

30. Kohlmeier L et al. 1997. Lycopene and myocardial infarction risk in the EURAMIC Study. *American Journal of Epidemiology* 146(8):618–626.

Street DA et al. 1994. Serum antioxidants and myocardial infarction. Are low levels of carotenoids and alpha-tocopherol risk factors for myocardial infarction? *Circulation* 90(3):1154–1161.

Su LC et al. 1998. Differences between plasma and adipose tissue biomarkers of carotenoids and tocopherols. *Cancer Epidemiology Biomarkers and Prevention* 7(11):1043–1048.

Agarwal S and Rao AV. 1998. Tomato lycopene and low density lipoprotein oxidation: a human dietary intervention study. *Lipids* 33(10):981–984.

Fuhrman B et al. 1997. Hypocholesterolemic effect of lycopene and beta–carotene is related to suppression of cholesterol synthesis and augmentation of LDL receptor activity in macrophages. *Biochemistry and Biophysiology Research Communications* 233:658–662.

31. Kontush A et al. 1997. Plasma ubiquinol-10 is decreased in patients with hyperlipidemia. *Atherosclerosis* 129(1):119–126.

Mortensen SA et al. 1997. Dose-related decrease of serum coenzyme Q10 during treatment with HMG-CoA reductase inhibitors. *Molecular Aspects of Medicine* 18(Suppl):S137–144.

Sing RB et al. 1999. Serum concentration of lipoprotein(a) decreases on treatment with hydrosoluble coenzyme Q10 in patients with coronary artery disease: discovery of a new role. *International Journal of Cardiology* 68(1):23–29.

Singh RB et al. 1998. Randomized, double-blind placebo-controlled trial of coenzyme Q10 in patients with acute myocardial infarction. *Cardiovascular Drug Therapy* 12(4):347–353.

32. Steiner M et al. 1996. A double-blind crossover study in moderately hypercholesterolemic men that compared the effect of aged garlic extract and placebo administration on blood lipids. *American Journal of Clinical Nutrition* 64(6):866–870.

Holzgartner H et al. 1992. Comparison of the efficacy and tolerance of a garlic preparation vs. bezafibrate. *Arzeimittelforschung* 42(12):1473–1477.

Bordia A. 1981. Effects of garlic on blood lipids in patients with coronary heart disease. *American Journal of Clinical Nutrition* 34(10):2100–2103.

Bordia A et al. 1998. Effect of garlic *(Allium sativum)* on blood lipids, blood sugar, fibrinogen and fibrinolytic activity in patients with coronary artery disease. *Prostaglandins Leukotrienes and Essential Fatty Acids* 58(4):257–263.

Ide N and Lau BH. 1999. Aged garlic extract attenuates intracellular oxidative stress. *Phytomedicine* 6(2):125–131.

Ide N and BH Lau. 1997. Garlic compounds protect vascular endothelial cells from oxidized low-density lipoprotein-induced injury. *Journal of Pharmacy and Pharmacology* 49(9):908–911.

Song K and J Milner. 1999. Heating garlic inhibits its ability to suppress 7,12-dimethylbenz(a) anthracene-induced DNA adduct formation in rat mammary tissue. *Journal of Nutrition* 129(3):657–661.

33. Singh RB *et al.* 1994. Hypolipidemic and antioxidant effects of *Commiphora mukul* as an adjunct to dietary therapy in patients with hypercholesterolemia. *Cardiovascular Drug Therapy* 8(4):659–664.

10

1. Tavassoli FA. 1997. The influence of endogenous and exogenous reproductive hormones on the mammary glands with emphasis on experimental studies in rhesus monkeys. *Verh Dtsch Ges Pathol* 81:514–520.

    Gapstur SM *et al.* 1999. Hormone replacement therapy and the risk of breast cancer with a favorable histology: results of the Iowa Women's Health Study. *Journal of the American Medical Association* 281(22):2091–1097.

2. Miller AB *et al.* 1997. The Canadian National Breast Screening Study: update on breast cancer mortality. *Journal of National Cancer Institute Monograms* 22:37–41.

3. World Cancer Research Fund/American Institute for Cancer Research. 1997. *Food, Nutrition and the Prevention of Cancer: a Global Perspective* Washington DC: American Institute for Cancer Research.

4. Hursting SD *et al.* 1990. Types of dietary fat and the incidence of cancer at 5 sites. *Preventative Medicine* 19:242–253.

    Rose DP *et al.* 1986. International comparisons of mortality rates for cancer of the breast, ovary, prostate and colon and per capita food consumption. *Cancer* 58:2263–2271.

    Woods MN *et al.* 1989. Low fat, high fibre diet and serum estrone sulfate in premenopausal women. *American Journal of Clinical Nutrition* 49:1179–1193.

    Prentice RL *et al.* 1988. Aspects of the rationale for the Women's Health Trial. *Journal of the National Cancer Institute* 80:802–814.

5. Boyd NF *et al.* A meta-analysis of studies of dietary-fat and breast cancer risk. *British Journal of Cancer* 68:627–636.

    Holmes MD *et al.* Association of dietary fat and fatty acids with risk of breast cancer. *Journal of the American Medical Association* 281(10): 914–920.

    Wu AH *et al.* 1999. Meta-analysis: dietary fat intake, serum estrogen levels, and the risk of breast cancer. *Journal of the National Cancer Institute.* 91(6):520–34.

6. Boyd NF *et al.* 1997. Effects at two years of a low fat, high carbohydrate diet on radiologic features of the breast: results from a randomized trial. Canadian Diet and Breast Cancer Prevention Study Group. *Journal of the National Cancer Institute* 89(7):488–496.

    Boyd NF *et al.* Effects of a low fat, high carbohydrate diet on plasma sex hormones in premenopausal women: results from a randomized trial. Canadian Diet and Breast Cancer Prevention Study Group. *British Journal of Cancer Institute* 76(1):127–135.

7. Zheng W *et al.* 1998. Well-done meat intake and the risk of breast cancer. *Journal of the National Cancer Institute* 90(22):1724–1729.

8. Knept P *et al.* Intake of dairy products and the risk of breast cancer. *British Journal of Cancer* 73(5):687–691.

    Ip MM *et al.* 1999. Conjugated linoleic acid inhibits proliferation and induces apoptosis of normal rat mammary epithelial cells in primary culture. *Experimental Cellular Research* 250(1):22–34.

    Thompson H *et al.* 1997. Morphological and biochemical status of the mammary glands as influenced by conjugated linoleic acid: implication for a reduction in mammary cancer risk. *Cancer Research* 57(22):5067–5072.

9. Rose DP *et al.* 1996. Effect of omega-3 fatty acids on the progression of metastases after surgical excision of human breast cancer cell solid tumors growing in nude mice. *Clinical Cancer Research* 2(10):1751–1756.

10. La Vecchia C *et al.* 1995. Olive oil, other dietary fats, and the risk of breast cancer (Italy). *Cancer Causes and Control* 6(6):545–550.

11. Lu LJ *et al.* 1996. Effects of soya consumption for one month on steroid hormones in premenopausal women: implications for breast cancer risk. *Cancer Epidemiology Biomarkers and Prevention* 5(1):63–70.

    Woods, M, 1999. Dietary soy supplement and menopausal hormones and hot flashes. Tufts University, Boston, Massachusetts. Abstract. Third International Symposium on Soy Foods in Treating and Preventing Chronic Disease.

    Cassidy A *et al.* 1993. Biological effects of plant oestrogens in premenopausal women. *FASEB Journal* 7:A866.

12. Li D *et al.* 1999. Soybean isoflavones reduce experimental metastasis in mice. *Journal of Nutrition* 129(5):1075–1078.

Shao ZM *et al.* 1998. Genistein exerts multiple suppressive effects on human breast carcinoma cells. *Cancer Research* 58(21):4851–4857.

Barnes S. 1997. The chemopreventative properties of soy isoflavonoids in animal models of breast cancer. *Breast Cancer Research and Treatment* 46(2-3):169–179.

Hsieh CY *et al.* 1998. Estrogenic effects of genistein on the growth of estrogen receptor-positive human breast cancer (MCF-7) cells in vitro and in vivo. *Cancer Research* 58(17):3833–3838.

13. McMichal-Phillips DF *et al.* 1998. Effects of soy-protein supplementation on epithelial proliferation in the histologically normal human breast. *American Journal of Clinical Nutrition* 68(6 Suppl):1431S–1435S.

14. Thompson LU *et al.* 1996. Flaxseed and its lignan and oil components reduce mammary tumor growth at a late stage of carcinogenesis. *Carcinogenesis* 17(6):1373–1376.

Thompson LU *et al.* 1996. Antitumorigenic effect of a mammalian lignan precurser from flaxseed. *Nutrition and Cancer* 26(2):159–165.

15. Hunter DJ *et al.* 1993. A prospective study of intake of vitamin C, E and A and the risk of breast cancer. *New England Journal of Medicine* 329:234–240.

Freudenheim JL *et al.* 1996. Premenopausal breast cancer risk and intake of vegetables, fruits and related nutrients. *Journal of the National Cancer Institute* 88(6):340–348.

16. Howe GR *et al.* 1990. Dietary factors and risk of breast cancer: combined analysis of 12 case-control studies. *Journal of the National Cancer Institute* 82:561–569.

Bagga D *et al.* 1995. Effects of a very low fat, high fibre diet in serum hormones and menstrual function. Implications for breast cancer prevention. *Cancer* 76(12):2491–2496.

Rose DP *et al.* 1997. Effects of diet supplementation with wheat bran on serum estrogen levels in the follicular and luteal phases of the menstrual cycle. *Nutrition* 13(6):535–539.

17. Van't Veer P *et al.* 1989. Consumption of fermented milk products and breast cancer: a case-control study in The Netherlands. *Cancer Research* 49(14):4020–4023.

Biffi A *et al.* 1997. Antiproliferative effect of fermented milk on the growth of a human breast cancer cell line. *Nutrition and Cancer* 28(1):93–99.

18. Hunter DJ *et al.* 1992. A prospective study of caffeine, coffee, tea and breast cancer. *American Journal of Epidemiology* 136:1000–1001 (Abstract).

Rogers AE *et al.* 1998. Black tea and mammary gland carcinogenesis by 7,12–dimethylbenz[a]anthracene in rats fed control or high fat diets. *Carcinogenesis* 19(7):1269–1273.

Weisburger JH *et al.* 1997. Tea, or tea and milk, inhibit mammary gland and colon carcinogenesis in rats. *Cancer Letter* 114(1–2):323–327.

Nakachi K *et al.* 1998. Influence of drinking green tea on breast cancer malignancy among Japanese patients. *Japanese Journal of Cancer Research* 89(3):254–261.

19. Cao G *et al.* Antioxidant capacity of tea and common vegetables. *Journal of Agriculture and Food Chemistry* 44(11):3426–3431.

20. Longnecker MP *et al.* 1994. Alcoholic beverage consumption in relation to risk of breast cancer: meta analysis and review. *Cancer Causes and Control* 5:73–82.

Hankinson SE *et al.* 1995. Alcohol, height, and adiposity in relation to estrogen and prolactin levels in postmenopausal women. *Journal of the National Cancer Institute* 87(17):1297–1302.

21. Hirose K *et al.* 1999. Effect of body size on breast cancer risk among Japanese women. *International Journal of Cancer* 80(3):349–355.

Huang Z *et al.* 1997. Dual effects of weight and weight gain on breast cancer risk. *Journal of the American Medical Association* 278(17):1407–1411.

La Vecchia C *et al.* 1997. Body mass index and post-menopausal breast cancer: an age-specific analysis. *British Journal of Cancer* 75(3):441–444.

22. Rohan TE *et al.* 1993. Dietary fibre, vitamins A, C, and E and the risk of breast cancer: a cohort study. *Cancer Causes and Control* 4:29–37.

Jain M and AB Miller. 1994. Premorbid diet and the prognosis of women with breast cancer. *Journal of the National Cancer Institute* 86(18):1390–1397.

Zhang S *et al.* 1999. Dietary carotenoids and vitamins A, C, and E and risk of breast cancer. *Journal of the National Cancer Institute* 91(6):547–556.

Rock CL *et al.* 1996. Carotenoids, vitamin A, and estrogen receptor status in breast cancer. *Nutrition and Cancer* 25(3):281–296.

23. Howe GR *et al.* 1990. Dietary factors and risk of breast cancer: combined analysis of 12 case-control studies. *Journal of the National Cancer Institute* 82:561–569

24. Wu K *et al.* 1999. A prospective study on folate, B12, and pyridoxal-5'-phosphate (B6) and breast cancer. *Cancer Epidemiology Biomarkers and Prevention* 8(3):209–217.

25. Zhang S *et al.* 1999. A prospective study of folate intake and the risk of breast cancer. *Journal of the American Medical Association* 281(17):1632–1637.

index